detox and revitalize

The Holistic Guide for Renewing Your Body, Mind, and Spirit

Susana L. Belen

Founder of *We Care*
Holistic Health Center

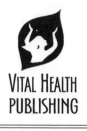

VITAL HEALTH
PUBLISHING

Danbury, CT

Detox and Revitalize: The Holistic Guide for Renewing Your Body, Mind, and Spirit

Published in 2005 by Vital Health Publishing, Danbury, CT

First Edition Copyright © Susana L. Belen 2005

Some content of this book was previously published under
Healthy Living: A Holistic Guide to Cleansing, Revitalization and Nutrition
First Edition Copyright © Susana Lombardi 1997
Second Edition Copyright © Susana Lombardi 2002

Cover Design: On the Dot Designs
Interior Book Design: Cathy Lombardi

Published by: Vital Health Publishing
      34 Mill Plain Road
      Danbury, CT 06811
      Office phone: 203-794-1009; Orders: 877-VIT-BOOKS
      Web site: www.vitalhealthbooks.com
      E-mail: info@vitalhealthbooks.com

Author Info: We Care Holistic Health Center
      18000 Long Canyon Rd.
      Desert Hot Springs, CA 92241
      760-251-2261 or 800-888-2523
      Web site: www.wecarespa.com

Notice of Rights
All rights reserved. No portion of this book may be reproduced or transmitted in any form or by any means, electronic, mechanical, photocopying, recording or otherwise, without the prior written permission of the publisher.

Disclaimer
Serious diseases should always be treated under medical supervision. There should be no delay in seeking medical advice if you have any persisting medical or psychological condition. The material in this book is for educational purposes only and is not intended for use in diagnosing or treating any individual.

Printed in the United States of America
ISBN: 1-890612-46-4

CONTENTS

PREFACE

Modern science and medicine have achieved great advances in understanding the molecular basis of life. Technological advances have allowed us to provide people with medications and surgical procedures that prolong life and relieve symptoms.
Yet even the latest discoveries can only support the body's reliance on its own inherent intelligence to reconstruct its functioning.

Our cells are alive: They breathe, take in nutrients, manufacture all kinds of substances, eliminate waste and toxic products, and also reproduce. All these processes consume energy.

When we eat we are putting our organism to work. Every aspect of eating consumes energy: We think about food, buy it, prepare it, cook it, chew, swallow, digest, absorb and assimilate it, and eliminate the waste. Every single cell of our body engages in some kind of work. Even though we generally think of food as our source of energy, the reality is that a great amount of energy—highly intelligent energy—is used every time we eat.

Our modern societies have invented all kinds of substances to preserve color and give fragrance to the foods we consume, as well as give them the flavors that will satisfy our increasingly sophisticated tastes. All these laboratory chemicals put a strain on the body's work of digestion and assimilation. Some of these substances cannot be processed by the cells and therefore accumulate as toxins and waste.

Curiously, medicine has somehow ignored these problems and is constantly inventing new substances and procedures to counteract and relieve their symptoms. Antacids are a typical example. These medications are dispensed so that people can continue to insult their organism with poor food choices (which cause the problems in the first place).

We observe that in nature, when animals get sick, they stop eating. Most diseases reduce our appetite as well. These are strong indications of a natural way the body uses to heal.

When we fast, we relieve our cells and major organs of arduous work. This *freed-up* energy becomes available for our organism to use in other processes that may have been put on *standby*. The elimination of waste reduces the toxic load and allows the cells to focus on repair and regeneration.

As a cardiologist, I am always on the lookout for healing tools. Fasting, which combines naturally with detoxification, is one of the most powerful tools I have found. Fasting boosts our inherent ability to heal without side effects and with very little risk.

Susana's health-care program is safe and enjoys the benefits of the research she has conducted over the past 20 years. In my four years of work at We Care, I have witnessed results in the realm of the miraculous. Weight loss, skin clearing, focused minds, and open hearts are just some of the effects. Conditions such as high blood pressure, high cholesterol, cancer, and other diseases have improved and healed right in front of my eyes.

It is with honor and great enthusiasm that I endorse Susana's work. It is my wish that the knowledge contained in this book, which is so much needed today, be made widely available to our world.

Alejandro Junger, M.D., F.A.C.C.
(310) 473-3888
2001 S. Barrington Ave., Suite # 101
Los Angeles, CA 90025

INTRODUCTION

why this book?

Over the past two decades, I have had extensive exposure to many aspects of the health field and, in recent years, have often been asked to compile a summary guide for a detoxification and revitalization program.

The intention of this concise book is to present basic principles of good eating and self-health care, providing a comprehensive survey helpful to the newcomer and of interest also to those with good previous nutritional background.

This handbook summarizes years of dedicated study of the work of many holistic health educators and practitioners. I am very grateful to have had the opportunity to benefit from their work. My own varied background in the health field—as a Hatha Yoga instructor, certified lymphologist, holistic practitioner, massage and colon therapist, and director and founder of We Care Holistic Health Center—has enabled me to include a number of tips and techniques not ordinarily found in nutritional sources.

The program described here will seldom conflict with any other therapy or treatment; however, if you are under a doctor's care, it is best to discuss this program and seek his or her counsel and support. Our program is not intended to supplant qualified health care. Not everyone needs this program, and we are not recommending it as a panacea. But there are many who will benefit from it.

Note: If you suffer from a bleeding bowel or any severe bowel disturbance, it is imperative that your doctor supervise your participation in this program.

my story

About 20 years ago I experienced some major challenges in my life. I was getting a divorce after many years of marriage and my situation was extremely precarious. I had four children to care for, no family members in this country, no profession, and almost no knowledge of the English language. I went into a panic. My emotional tension was so severe that my bowels stopped moving and I became very constipated. In my search for help, I was fortunate to find a local chiropractor who taught me how to cleanse with juices and gave me a colonic every day. Under his care I made an amazing recovery. By the end of only the second week, I had become a totally different person. Instead of weeping and yelling uncontrollably, I found myself able to speak and listen calmly to my friends and family.

The transformation in my personality was so drastic that I thought to myself, "Fasting is magical—I need to find out more about this." Led by my curiosity, I began reading any books on the subject I could get my hands on and taking classes and workshops. Gradually I developed the knowledge and skill to become a vegetarian, a yoga instructor, a massage and colon therapist, a certified lymphologist, and a transformational breath instructor.

The more I learned, the more excited I became about putting all this new knowledge into practice in my life. My enthusiasm inspired my friends to know more about a healthier way of life, and they began to organize talks for me to give in their homes to groups of five to ten people. Within a short time, I began to receive letters from the participants thanking me for their improved sense of health and well-being, and expressing appreciation for all they had learned. Many of these people encouraged me to open a place where I could teach them more. One day when I was reading these letters, I decided that opening a health center was truly the way for me to make my best contribution to mankind. At such a center, I could focus on sharing my small knowledge on how to live life without aches and pains, and without medications and drugs such as antidepressants.

The information contained in this book comes from my heart with the desire to help you become happier and healthier through detoxing and revitalizing practices. I present here what I believe and what I practice every day of my life. I pray that this information will help you achieve the same results I have experienced.

—Susana L. Belen

*"The doctor of the future will give no medicine
but will interest his patient in the care of the human frame,
in diet and in the cause and prevention of disease."*

—Thomas A. Edison

To the Reader:

The information in this book should not be interpreted or represented as a claim for cure, diagnosis, treatment, or prevention of any disease or condition. It should be used only as educational information about utilizing nature's way of living. The concepts included here have been practiced by thousands of people throughout the world as an alternative way of looking at the life process. Do not embark on any health regimen without consultation and approval by your doctor or health practitioner.

PART I

Cleansing
Revitalization
and
Nutrition

The more you cleanse,

the fewer cravings you will have,

and the easier it will be

to stay on a more healthful diet.

1 why detox and revitalize your body?

If you have picked up this book because you want to lose a few pounds and look better, my advice is to close the book now. You will save time and be happier if you join a health club, exercise a little, tone your muscles, and just look great. Following the instructions printed here takes understanding, commitment, and effort. Only when your motivation is strong will you want to embrace and follow the process described in this book.

Let me explain. When an animal becomes sick in the jungle, does it need to go to a veterinarian? No. It will rest, not eat for a while, and then be guided by instinct to the specific food that will save its life. Believe it or not, you were born with this same instinct, but you have lost touch with it. When? Each time you turn on the television or read magazines, books, and newspapers that tell you what to do, what to buy, what to eat, or what is good for you.

Why is it so easy to accept and follow all these suggestions? Because our bodies and minds have grown numb from all the chemicals in the foods we eat each day—artificial colorings, artificial flavorings, preservatives, synthetic foods, genetically engineered foods, salt, sugar. Our bodies do not digest or eliminate these chemicals, so they accumulate in our fluids and tissues. Over time we become more lethargic, we have less energy, we catch more colds and flus. Perhaps we consider these changes signs of *old age*, but they are actually symptoms of toxification.

If you eat the foods and follow the lifestyle of the majority of the population in the United States, you have a 50 percent chance of contracting a major disease such as cancer, arthritis, arteriosclerosis, heart disease, diabetes, or AIDS. Children today are born with conditions that only 10 years ago were considered diseases of old age; more children under the age of 11 are dying of cancer and diabetes than any other diseases.

So what can you do? Learn to take care of yourself and protect yourself from environmental and food pollution. Learn how your body and mind work. Learn how to detoxify—to remove all those chemicals that have accumulated in your fluids and tissues—and let your body begin to regenerate itself. Yes, your body has the power to regenerate itself! Every minute of your life millions of cells are dying and millions more are being reborn. Your body creates 2.5 billion red blood cells per second. Within 11 months, not one single cell that is in your body today will still be there (except for brain cells). Next year you will have a brand new body. So how do you want your body to be? A little sicker and older, or healthier and stronger?

Strong healthy cells are what make a body strong. How do you help create strong healthy cells? The key lies in the foods you put in your mouth, the thoughts you put in your head, and the feelings you place in your heart. Together, these feed the blood that travels 60,000 miles within your body—three times the circumference of the earth—carrying physical strength and mental and emotional power to every cell. If you want to be a healthier, happier person, you want to make sure that every spoonful of food you bring to your mouth is the highest quality possible. You want to foster thoughts and feelings that are loving and caring.

As you begin to observe how you feel when you improve your diet, control your thoughts, and foster peaceful feelings, you will know what to do and what not to do. You will become *your own doctor*, truly able to support your right to be healthy. You will know that the only reason you want to detoxify your body and eat organic whole foods is because then and only then can your inner guidance lead you to the right foods, the right job, the right companion, and everything you deserve.

suggested reading

Nestle, Marion
Food Politics
University of California Press, Berkeley, CA, 2003

Fox, Nicols
Spoiled
Basic Books, A Division of Harper Collins Publishers,
New York, NY, 1998

Trudeau, Kevin
Natural Cures They Don't Want You to Know About
Alliance Publishing Group, Hensdale, IL, 2004

2 five principles of balanced health

THE FACTS

The U.S. Public Health Service has reported the rate of health deterioration among the American people. Out of the 100 nations included in their survey, America was the healthiest in 1900. By 1920, we had dropped to the second-healthiest nation. During World War II, we went back to number one—that's when sugar and meat were hard to get and family vegetable gardens were common. By 1978, we had dropped to seventy-ninth. In 1980, we were ninety-fifth. We have now hit rock bottom—that's number 100 on the list! Yet we are said to be the wealthiest nation in the world. Who or what is responsible?

A DEPARTURE FROM NATURE

The basic, sensible theories of health care that prevailed in 1900 have changed dramatically over the past century. The major change has been the shift from nature—or natural healing methods—to drugs. Accompanying this shift has been the increasing use of preservatives and chemicals and our exposure to them in food, polluted air, and synthetic fabrics. This unnatural approach to life has had a detrimental effect on the American people. In my opinion, as long as our approach to healing (except in rare cases) involves the use of drugs, chemicals, radiation, and scalpels, we will never be truly well. If we sincerely want to restore the American people to health, or if we personally wish to reclaim our own individual health, we must return to God and follow his ways—Mother Nature's ways—by using herbs and other natural methods that purify and strengthen the body.

THE FOUNTAIN OF YOUTH

We all wish for a simple, mystical, magical something that will completely free our bodies from the discomfort of illness or the infirmities of old age.

Every generation in every civilization throughout recorded history has sought after a fountain of youth, in one form or another. Can you imagine a pearl of such great price? To enjoy a body that would stabilize at the point of maturity and never succumb to the commonly accepted course of degeneration that we call *disease* or *the aging process*. Down through the ages, many have dreamt of discovering magical waters or a kind of food—a vitamin, a mineral, a drug—or perhaps a secret substance that would make eternal youth a reality.

Over the past decade, our hopes have dimmed. Our enthusiastic anticipation of such a dream come true has been all but destroyed as we have observed the most advanced medical technology in history assume near total authority over our health, while at the same time failing to reduce the power of disease.

We witness the death of our children from diseases that only 10 years ago would have been called diseases of old age. And what hope are we given when our doctors are dying of the same degenerative diseases that afflict millions of people right now in our own country?

Since we have little choice but to preoccupy ourselves with mere survival—with arresting the process of degeneration and doing whatever we can to avoid developing a degenerative disease—how can we sustain the twin hopes of ending the nightmare of disease and stopping the aging process as well?

If I didn't feel very confident that I have a logical solution to share with you, I would never want to focus your attention so powerfully on the dreary realities of our present health status in the United States. Even so, I do not believe that anyone will ever discover any one substance that can halt the processes of degeneration and aging. Why? Because I believe that the secret to ageless, disease-free, balanced, and vibrant good health lies within *five principles of balanced health*. By following them, you can replace degeneration and aging with regeneration and ever-increasing vitality. Before discussing the five principles, however, I would like to shed some light on the way degeneration takes place.

THE PROCESS OF DEGENERATION

Why do we eat food? Besides pleasure, there is only one reason—to provide the building blocks needed to replace the cells being destroyed by what we call *aging* or *degenerative disease*. These terms are synonymous and describe the same process. Each gives a different perspective on the same condition: premature cell destruction in the body. The body's need for nutrition always reflects the level of cell destruction occurring in the body. This is of the utmost importance, for if we have the option of choosing to eat foods that stop premature cell destruction, we can make this our goal. If there is no premature cell destruction, there is no aging, and therefore no degeneration. That is logical enough, isn't it?

Centuries ago human beings survived, for the most part, by eating meat. Our ancestors discovered that cooking meat improved its flavor. As time passed, the cooking of food became a way of life and, for many, a great art. Today, nearly all of our food is cooked before it is eaten.

reviewing the process of degeneration

At best, raw foods contain from 5 to 75 percent of the enzymes needed for the process of digestion. Although the current popular trend is toward eating more raw foods, our raw fruits and vegetables today are as deficient in minerals and enzymes as cooked vegetables in the past, because of modern farming methods. Any form of processing, such as cooking, reduces these already low enzyme levels drastically.

This may not seem like a real threat, since it is widely believed that "the body is meant to digest the food; the food isn't supposed to digest itself." The live enzymes in raw food, however, are meant to assist the body in the process of digestion. Cooked food does not contain these enzymes, so when we eat cooked food, the body has to sacrifice its metabolic enzymes—the life force of the body—for the process of digestion. *This sacrificing of metabolic enzymes is the fundamental physical cause of the aging process and the process of degeneration.*

A second, closely related problem is the habit of consuming larger quantities of food than the body is capable of digesting and assimilating. These two practices—cooking and overeating—together cause a toxic buildup of undigested food residues in the colon. As a result, harmful bacteria and fungus multiply in the bowel, and the body loses vitality as it struggles to neutralize these damaging elements.

While undigested food residues are putrefying in the colon, excess waste material overloads other systems of the body as well. As a result of poor fat digestion, for example, the arteries become clogged. This happens when the natural lipase enzymes and essential fatty acids in fats and oils are overheated and destroyed in cooking. Without these cofactors, the body cannot produce enough lecithin to break down and properly utilize cholesterol or fats. The result is a buildup of unusable, solid fatty fuel that clogs the arteries, restricting circulation—our fueling system—and contributing to the development of heart disease, stroke, and all circulatory disorders.

When digestion is poor, the proper nutrients are not delivered to the cells, and nutritional deficiencies and metabolic imbalances develop throughout the body. Since there is more toxic waste than the organs of elimination can handle, tissue cells are constantly being destroyed at a very rapid rate. When we add to all of this the clogging up of the skin and the backing up of the lymphatic system, we have a body tragically and unnecessarily afflicted by the aging process and the process of degeneration. This is the unfortunate condition of the average American adult body.

Having identified the problem, we can now proceed with a discussion of the solution. The following is adapted with permission from *The Five Principles of Balanced Health*, a book by Dr. Mick Hall.

FIRST PRINCIPLE—DETOXIFICATION AND BALANCE

We have five organs of elimination: the colon, skin, lungs, liver, and kidneys. We also have two complete systems that play key roles in detoxifying the body: the circulatory and lymphatic systems. These organs and systems are intended to keep the body disease-free and operating at maximum efficiency. With so many avenues for the elimination of bodily waste, we might assume that our bodies are well equipped to handle the accumulations that poison our cells. Unfortunately, so many environmental conditions and misguided practices undermine our health that our organs and systems of elimination are too stressed and overwhelmed to keep up with the toxic load. Therefore, we now have a choice: pay the consequences, or learn how to detoxify and balance our bodies.

detoxification

To begin the process of detoxification, we need to start with the colon, the skin, and the lungs.

colon. The colon is literally the garbage can of the body. If we do not empty the kitchen garbage can for a few days, the bacterial activity in the garbage produces an offensive odor, and unwelcome insects are drawn to the smorgasbord to dine. A similar condition is found in at least 90 percent of the colons in America. I am not implying that most people do not have a bowel movement every day. I mean that today's elimination isn't always yesterday's waste. It may be from at least the day before yesterday. Any tube or pipe that constantly carries decomposing food and body waste accumulates a buildup on its walls. This buildup begins when we are children, shortly after cooked foods are introduced into our diet, and continues to accumulate thereafter.

It has been estimated that 90 percent of the U.S. population has parasites. Given that almost every colon provides the perfect environment for parasitic life, this estimate is probably conservative.

There are two solutions to this problem: The first is to clear the colon wall completely of the accumulated waste buildup, and the second is to balance the flora within the colon. For the best methods of properly cleansing the colon, see Chapter 3, "Colon Detoxification." The balancing of the intestinal flora will be dealt with in the next section of this chapter entitled "Balance."

skin. The skin is the largest organ of elimination. Second to the bowel, the skin eliminates more waste than any other organ. Because a sedentary lifestyle is so common today, most people lose the tremendous benefit of the large volume of waste that could be eliminated through the skin. When the skin fails to handle its own workload, the burden must be shared by the other organs of elimination.

Of course, the most natural methods of stimulating the skin are physical labor, exercise, and active recreation. Methods such as dry skin brushing, scrubbing showers, herbal glow treatments, and cleansing baths also help the skin eliminate accumulated waste. It would be beneficial to follow the instructions for the cleansing bath most appropriate for your needs. Find these instructions in the section "Detoxifying Baths" on page 19.

lungs. The lungs not only eliminate large amounts of carbon dioxide, but also supply us with a generous amount of oxygen. It is important for our health to keep the lungs clean and able to exchange as large a volume of air as possible. Consider the difference between a wood stove with the draft open wide, allowing a large volume of oxygen into the firebox and thus creating a powerful, hot fire, and a similar stove with the draft nearly closed, the fire barely able to maintain a flame. Oxygen is just as vital to our energy production as it is to the fire. Yet the lungs cannot perform to the best of their ability when day after day we breathe shallowly and hardly expel all the old air. To keep our lung capacity high, we need to use our lungs properly, through practicing deep-breathing exercises, sports, and/or general aerobic exercise. The following method of detoxifying the lymphatic system is also of great benefit to the respiratory system.

lymphatic system. Detoxifying the lymphatic system is important to the health of tissue cells as well as to all-around body hygiene. The lymphatic system carries blood proteins and cell waste away from tissue cells to prevent the cells from being poisoned in their own waste. When we aren't active enough, the lymphatic system slows down and doesn't properly clear the tissue of this waste. A sluggish lymphatic system allows toxic fluids to remain in the body longer than necessary. This causes these fluids to become more toxic, and the body to dissipate its vital energy in protecting itself from these toxins. A sluggish lymphatic system also restricts cell function by limiting the effectiveness of oxygen. There are two effective ways to detoxify the lymphatic system. The first is the detox bath (see instructions in the section "Detoxifying Baths," p. 19). The second is the lymphatic exercise of bouncing on a small, round trampoline.

balance

There are three important areas in creating balance: pH, bacteria, and minerals.

pH balancing and digestion. There are three body fluids that provide us with information regarding the environment or state of the body chemistry: the blood, urine, and saliva. The kidneys are constantly filtering the blood and regulating the body chemistry to maintain a proper pH. This is achieved by the kidneys continually eliminating all mineral excesses. In this way, the chemistry in the blood is being constantly altered according to the added influences of the diet, digestion, and other metabolic processes. This important regulating function of the kidneys makes it possible for the blood to maintain a constant 7.4 pH (potential of Hydrogen). A 7.4 pH is essential for proper digestion to occur.

The body's ability to maintain a proper pH is determined by proper digestion, and the key to proper digestion is determined by proper pH. If this seems to you like a *catch 22*, you're right! When proteins are properly digested, sufficient hydrogen is released, allowing the body to produce hydrochloric acid. With sufficient hydrochloric acid, complete protein digestion can occur. When carbohydrates are properly digested, sufficient bicarbonates are released, which join with the organic form of sodium to neutralize the acids and balance the pH. Without these acids being neutralized, they can threaten to reduce the pH of the blood. It places a tremendous stress on the whole system if the pH is raised or reduced by even 0.2 pH. It is vital for the body to maintain a close tolerance to the 7.4 pH. This is the key to proper digestion, as well as sustaining life itself within the body.

If a person has a habit of eating an excessive amount of acid-forming foods, the pH will tend toward being too acidic, which inhibits proper digestion. This becomes serious when the same individual is incapable of digesting complex carbohydrates. This is due to the fact that there is an excess intake of acid-forming proteins causing a loss of phosphorus, the mineral needed for carbohydrate metabolism, thereby inhibiting the long-term digestion of carbohydrates. Digestion is imperative. Proper digestion releases the nutrients needed to regulate and balance all body functions. If digestion is inhibited in any form, the undigested food becomes toxic waste within the intestinal tract, and eventually the blood. The body's ability to function properly and complete all necessary metabolic processes is also hindered.

It is easy to see why improving digestion is a critical factor in the body's ability to maintain a proper pH, thereby ensuring proper digestion. Research has found that the most effective way of improving digestion, and thereby balancing the fluid pH, is by the use of concentrated plant enzymes.

balancing bacteria. Balancing the bacteria or intestinal flora of the colon is just as important as cleansing the colon wall. There are literally hundreds of different types of bacteria in the bowel. Some are friendly, and some are destructive to our health. The balance should be maintained at approximately 85 percent friendly bacteria to 15 percent harmful bacteria. Unfortunately, in many people, this ratio is close to being just the opposite. In this unbalanced state, the colon becomes a generator of harmful, disease-producing bacteria and fungus, creating an environment hospitable to the development of more serious disease conditions.

Dr. Paul Gyorgy (who discovered vitamin B_6) has determined that the main component of normal human intestinal flora is *lactobacillus bifidus*. This bacterium establishes itself in the colons of newborns when they are fed mother's milk; it is found in the nipples of lactating mothers. This is why the use of bifidus in the rebalancing process is so important. Two effective methods of reintroducing bifidus into the body involve oral intake and retention enemas. You will find instructions for oral use of bifidus on page 34 and instructions for retention enemas on page 19.

balancing minerals. If minerals are not in the proper balance, radiant health is an elusive dream. Space limitation makes it impossible to do justice here to the subject of minerals. Suffice it to say that a daily intake of chlorophyll, goat's whey, and chelated minerals will provide a good daily balance of minerals. Also, eliminating sugar from the diet will reduce the loss of calcium. For more on these recommendations, read the "Average Day's Diet" in Chapter 8 (pp. 52–53).

SECOND PRINCIPLE—NUTRITION

It is not what you eat but what you digest and assimilate that nourishes the body.

Nutrition is a controversial subject today. Most people who become interested in nutrition soon find themselves prey to two silent fears: the fear of eating and the fear of not eating. This applies to supplements as well as foods: Without clear knowledge of what the body needs, determining which supplements to take and in what quantities can become a dangerous guessing game we play at our own risk. My own research suggests that nutrition can cause as many health problems as it solves.

There seem to be three major types of problems. The first, and most common, is *over-supplementing*. Nutritional supplements and herbal combinations have become a big business, and the average person needs guidance in establishing a reasonable program of supplementation. It is wonderful that we have the freedom to care for our individual needs as we see fit. Of course we need to be concerned with the quality of our supplements, but we also need to realize how concentrated these supplemental tablets and capsules are. The average health program recommends at least three times more supplementation than the body can assimilate. The body is then incapable of eliminating the supplements quickly enough, and the vitamins intended to nourish us contribute to toxicity instead. Dr. Mick Hall offers recommendations to readers regarding reasonable amounts of supplementation in his book *The Five Principles of Balanced Health*.

The second problem is the following of *special diets* geared to accomplishing a particular goal or bringing about a certain metabolic change. In most cases, the target is the elimination of some type of bodily condition. Whatever the desired end result, the simple need of the body to replace destroyed tissue cells is almost always overlooked.

The third area of concern is *personal eating habits*. The one common denominator among centenarians is the eating of small quantities of food. Everything we eat meets one of two fates: it is digested and used to nourish our bodies, or it is eliminated as a waste product in a process that robs us of energy. This is why we need to consider both the quality and the quantity of everything we eat. If a food doesn't contain elements that help to build our body, it should be passed over or taken in very small quantities.

I would like to share the results of an experiment to illustrate the seriousness of what I am pointing out here. Scientists used two similar groups of dogs for this experiment. To one group, they gave only water. To the other, they gave water and white bread. After 30 days, the group on the water was still strong and healthy. The dogs in the group that was given water and white bread all died within two weeks. Do we conclude from this that white bread is poisonous? Of course not. But again, everything we eat needs to be of high enough quality to be digested and become blood, or it must be eliminated as a waste product and thereby rob the body of vital energy. So what happened to the dogs? They became fatigued to death. Why? Because the white bread took more energy to eliminate than it provided as nourishment (Mick Hall, N.D., *The Five Principles of Balanced Health*). Through a similar process, the average American is constantly half-fatigued to death from overeating. "Oh, what's a little excess as long as it's good, wholesome, raw food," we may say. But does it really matter what the food is if the body has already had enough? Some foods are easier to eliminate than others, and some are less toxic than others, but if the supply exceeds the demand, the excess must be eliminated as waste. This process of eliminating the excess saps the body's vitality no matter what the food.

There are a few guidelines that I feel are important to keep in mind as you establish the nutritional program best suited to your personal needs. First of all, I believe that just as we have a spiritual belief system and a mental belief system, the body has its own belief system. Our bodies are built of elements derived from our family eating habits. Our particular pattern of eating has established a level of expectation within the body, and an abrupt change in eating patterns disturbs its functioning unnecessarily. Changes in diet should be made slowly. The body can handle doing without food much easier than it can adapt to drastic changes. Eliminating from the diet as many harmful substances as possible is the only quick change that should be made.

Conduct a careful analysis of your personal diet. If the following items are part of your daily regime, cut back and eventually eliminate them: canned meats, pork products, processed meats, processed cheese, heated oils, white sugar, white wheat flour, white rice, processed foods, fast foods, microwave meals, and canned vegetables.

Lemonade

Mix three ounces of freshly squeezed lemon juice into a pint of water and sweeten to taste with maple syrup (only if you are free of candida and hypoglycemia) or stevia. You may enjoy the healthy addition of a dash of cayenne pepper. Fresh lemonade will assist your body's morning cleansing cycle.

Next, be aware that the body goes through a natural cleansing cycle every day from approximately 4:00 A.M. to noon. It therefore conflicts with nature to force the body into a feeding cycle right in the middle of a cleansing cycle. If you are a determined breakfast person, try to satisfy your needs with fruit and a pint of lemonade until at least 11:00 A.M. before eating breakfast. The section "Average Day's Diet" in Chapter 8 will provide a clearer picture of what an average day should be like while you are following this program.

The next—and crucial—step in structuring a nutrition program is to include more raw fruits and vegetables. (Read Chapter 8 and the recipes in Part II for more help in developing a personal nutritional program.)

THIRD PRINCIPLE—DIGESTION

Poor digestion is the number one cause of all common health complaints. Almost no one in this country over 20 years old has proper digestion, even when there are no obvious symptoms of indigestion such as heartburn or gas. If you are not employing supplemental enzymes to digest food, or if at least 20 percent of your food is cooked, you have poor digestion.

The purpose of digestive enzymes excreted by the body is to help food enzymes break down the food. Your body was never meant to do all the digesting it has to do when you eat a completely cooked meal. To produce the digestive enzymes necessary for the work of digestion, the body must give up its own life force. To understand this better, let us look for a moment at the time of birth.

When a baby is born, it has what is called *a metabolic enzyme pool*. This enzyme pool can be added to or subtracted from, just like a bank account. If the baby nurses at its mother's breast, enzymes are added to the pool. If the baby isn't able to nurse, it loses this additional deposit into the enzyme pool and will suffer the consequences. This enzyme pool corresponds to the level of life force within the body and is directly inherited. If the parents' enzyme pool or life force is low, the child inherits a low level of life force. If the parents possess a healthy level of enzymes, the child inherits a high level of life force or enzyme pool. This is the major difference between a person who is basically quite robust and another who always seems to be frail or sickly.

The level of your enzyme pool and how you conserve these reserves determines the level of your health and the length of your life. It is very common to live life burning the candle at both ends up to the age of about 40. Then, all of a sudden it becomes a matter of survival to step on the brakes a little and make a few lifestyle and dietary changes. The body is sending a signal that the enzyme pool is being emptied far too fast: If serious changes aren't made soon, life will no longer be possible. When your enzyme pool is empty or, in other words, when your life force is gone, you die. Thus you are left with two areas of concern: to determine how to conserve your enzyme pool, and to replace the enzymes that have already been used up.

To conserve the enzymes you still possess, you need to stop using them. This can be accomplished by adopting a program to halt premature tissue destruction. How? By eating more raw fruits and vegetables. The final, but most powerful step, is to use the correct supplemental enzymes for your personal needs.

Adopting a program to stop premature tissue destruction will also help replace the enzymes you have already used. In the program presented in *The Five Principles of Balanced Health*, one important step is designed especially to enhance the replacement of the enzyme pool. This is the practice of drinking a pint of lemonade each morning. (See the lemonade recipe, p. 16.) The lemon is one of nature's most cleansing foods, especially when picked ripe. Lemon juice cleanses and stimulates the liver, activating its power to transform food and supplemental enzymes into metabolic enzymes to replace what has been consumed from the metabolic pool. So do yourself a great favor and follow this program as closely as possible. Enjoy the thrill of drinking from a real fountain of youth. You will experience a return to a level of health you thought was lost.

FOURTH PRINCIPLE—EXERCISE

Movement is life: the more movement, the more life. There are five systems of the body that need the stimulation of exercise: the lymphatic, circulatory, respiratory, organ, and muscular systems. In this program, exercise is necessary to assist in the process of detoxification, to tone all body tissues, to increase oxygen intake for energy, and to stimulate circulation for proper fueling of tissue cells.

I would encourage spending 10 minutes, three times a day, working out on a small, round trampoline. This is an ideal exercise. It helps clear the lymphatic system, stimulates the circulation, strengthens the heartbeat, satisfies the needs of the respiratory system, and tones every cell in the body. Using the mini-trampoline, taking brisk walks, and practicing daily yoga are the very best exercises.

FIFTH PRINCIPLE—FOCUSED ATTENTION

The fifth principle is my favorite and, I believe, the most important. Expanding on the scripture, James Allen wrote in his beautiful book *As A Man Thinketh*, "As a man thinketh in his heart, so is he." In this little book, Allen explains beautifully the process by which our daily thoughts solidify into the circumstances of our lives.

When we decide on a goal we want to achieve, we plan, work, dream, and finally attain the desired goal. At the time of achieving that desired goal, we are aware of the connection between our first thought of the goal and the circumstances of achieving it.

A simplified way of looking at the same process is to realize that "we always go where we are looking." Life tends to make our thoughts manifest by bringing about the circumstances that mirror our thoughts. If we focus unduly on externals, for example, whether objects or people, we transfer our personal power to them, and lose command of our power to direct our lives toward the fulfillment of our deepest inner desires. So be careful about the focus of your attention. Be sure you are focusing on where you want to go.

Stop and take careful note of your daily thoughts and words. Thoughts are things! Every thought or word that you find yourself repeating, even when you are joking, is busy creating your future circumstances. Remember: You always go where you are looking. Where are you looking? Are you sure that is where you want to go? Are you looking down the road of joy, health, happiness, love, and purpose? Is it easier for you to list your faults or your positive qualities? Do you find it easier to focus on the faults or the positive qualities of your friends and coworkers? I pose these questions simply to clarify the reason why it often seems that life could be a bit brighter.

I hope that in this program—instead of concentrating on health problems and treatments—you will focus your attention on joyfully getting on with your healthy, happy life.

I would like to challenge you to a daily activity that I believe will help you to focus your attention. Put one of the following titles on the top left side of a sheet of paper:

1. My favorite people
2. People who inspire me
3. Everything I am grateful for in life
4. Everything in life that makes me happy or that I like
5. Things I would like to do
6. Dreams I would like to achieve.

Then make your list under the title. You may want to choose more than one title. Work every day on completing these lists until you feel comfortable with what you have written. If you have a lot to say, a notebook may be more suitable. When your lists are complete, continue by reviewing them every morning and every evening. We always go where we are looking. Get excited and inspired by where the new focus of your attention is taking you.

detoxifying baths

detox bath (for general detoxification and for detoxifying radiation, chemicals, and pollutants from your body). Put one package or suggested amount of a detoxifying bath into a tub of warm water. Lie in the tub for 20 to 30 minutes and perspire. When finished, take a warm scrubbing shower. Finish the process with a cool shower. The cooler the water, the more energy you stimulate back into the body.

Detox baths often contain the following ingredients to draw toxins out of the body: natural mineral salts from ancient mineral ocean beds, sodium bicarbonate, bentonite clay, and powdered herbs.

Instructions
Before bathing, drink a hot tea and brush the skin to open the pores.

We highly recommend:
- We Care Detox Bath (available from www.wecarespa.com)
- Detox Spa (available from many online holistic stores)
- LL's Magnetic Detox Clay Baths (available from many online holistic stores).

clorox bath (for metal and chemical detoxification). Pour 1 cup of Clorox into a full tub of warm water. Lie in tub for 20 to 30 minutes. Take a scrubbing soapy shower after. You may wish to put lotion on your body when finished. *Caution:* ventilate bathroom well to avoid breathing the Clorox fumes; always avoid skin contact with undiluted Clorox.

apple cider vinegar bath (helps restore pH and can be used for radiation exposure). Add 2 cups of apple cider vinegar to a warm bath; soak 15–30 minutes.

retention enema

Every night while fasting, dissolve 5 capsules of acidophilus in 3 ounces of water. Absorb the water into a rectal syringe and, while lying in bed, empty the syringe into the rectum. The goal is not to evacuate the intestines but to keep the acidophilus liquid in as long as possible.

Tip: As long as you remain lying down, you should not experience any urgency to urinate or defecate. Even 20 minutes will be highly beneficial.

suggested reading

Allen, James
As A Man Thinketh
Devorss, 1979

Hall, Mick, N.D.
The Five Principles of Balanced Health
www.drmickhall.com
(date of publication N/A)

3 the seven most important steps for rejuvenation and well-being

STEP 1. AVOIDING TOXINS

Avoid External Pollution

1. Air. Use an air purification system.
2. Water. Do not drink tap water. Have your own home filter.
3. Cleaning supplies. Use white vinegar and other natural products. Be more concerned about the cleanliness of your lungs than the cleanliness of your windows! Remember that toxic chemicals in cleaning solutions are inhaled and absorbed through the skin.
4. Cosmetics. Avoid anything containing artificial fragrance.
5. In your food. Avoid artificial colorings and flavorings, preservatives, sulfites, nitrates, salt, and sugar. If you want to improve your well-being, your diet should consist of organic natural food that you prepare from scratch, such as fresh fruits, fresh vegetables, seeds, nuts, whole grains, and legumes. If you are semivegetarian, occasionally add free-range eggs and chicken without antibiotics or hormones.

Avoid Internal Pollution—DETOXIFY!

We have 75 trillion cells in our bodies. Every cell absorbs nutrients, performs combustion, and expels waste. The normal functioning of every cell produces waste that needs to be carried out through the five channels of elimination.

1. The lymphatic system. The lymphatic system is the vacuum cleaner of the body. It helps to eliminate toxins through up-and-down movement and breathing exercises. Jumping on a mini-trampoline, walking, practicing inverted yoga poses and deep yogic breathing, all assist the lymph system.
2. The kidneys. Our kidneys are the body's filters. Drink lots of fluids to wash away toxins.
3. The bowels. Be sure to have two bowel movements every day. Every disease begins in the colon.
4. The lungs. We expel carbonic acid from our lungs. Breathe deeply.
5. The skin. The largest organ of elimination is the surface of our skin. Brush your skin dry every day before showering. We are supposed to eliminate two pounds of toxins daily through the pores of the skin.

Undigested food residues, damaged cells, dead cells, and chemicals from our environment and foods constitute a source of internal pollution that needs to be eliminated.

STEP 2. ONE DAY OF CLEANSING

Incorporate the healthy practice of one day of cleansing each week into your lifestyle. On your day of cleansing, do not eat any solid food, but only drink fluids. The simplest way is to drink lemon water. Prepare the lemon water by squeezing the juice of four lemons into a half-gallon of pure water. Place this in a thermos and drink on an hourly basis throughout the day.

STEP 3. GOOD DIGESTION

Follow the rules of good digestion so your body can absorb all the nutrients it needs.
- Relax before your meal.
- Chew your food well.
- Drink no more than one cup or glass of liquid at mealtime.
- Eat only on an empty stomach. Eat two solid meals a day and drink nutritional drinks between those meals. The third meal can usually be converted to a liquid *smoothie* prepared in a blender.

STEP 4. BREATHING EXERCISES

Set up a time each day for breathing exercises. Oxygenate your body. Oxygen is the best fuel for your system.

STEP 5. KITCHEN ORGANIZATION

Learn to organize your kitchen so your "fast food" is prepared at home. What I call *fast foods* are foods that you can prepare ahead of time and serve within 10 minutes of arriving home. They include smoothies, salads, steamed veggies, and soups. Rice, beans, lentils, and pasta can be cooked in large enough quantities, divided into small portions, and kept frozen. Warming up your own homemade food can save lots of food preparation and cleaning time, while guaranteeing you tasty and nutritional food (see Chapter 8, p. 59.). Go out to eat occasionally, but only to the best restaurants where you know the owner or chef and can count on having high-quality food.

STEP 6. RELAXATION

Adopt a method of relaxation that seems agreeable to you, perhaps yoga, meditation, breathing, music, dancing, or a hobby. Most important, avoid becoming STRESSED! What makes you stressed out? Your thinking, especially when you worry. So learn to control your thinking. If you don't learn to control your thinking, your thinking will control you.

STEP 7. TRUST

Trust in yourself, trust in the universe, trust in the process. Otherwise, how can you be relaxed enough to gather the energy to make all these changes?

To illustrate what I mean by trust I would like to tell you a story from the life of Thomas Edison. When he was 65 years old, Edison was still conducting daily experiments, working in a huge plant worth $2 million. Since the plant was supposed to be fireproof, he had insured it for only $200,000. One day as he was coming to work, he saw that the whole building was on fire. He immediately called out to his assistant, "Go get my wife! She must see this blaze—there will never be another fire like this again!" Next he commented, "With this fire all my mistakes are gone." Two weeks later he discovered the phonograph and, not long afterward, rebuilt his plant.

We may not all be able to act so cool and calm under similar circumstances, but we each can know, from the bottom of our heart, that even if we have a rough time today, tomorrow things can be wonderful once again. After the storm, the sun shines, and the clouds disappear.

Taking care of yourself will make you healthy and happy, and that is the best contribution you can make to the universe.

suggested reading

Diamond, John, M.D.
Facets of a Diamond: Reflections of a Healer
Enhancement Books, Danbury, CT, 2003

Khalsa, Dharma Singh, M.D.
Food as Medicine
Atria Books, New York, NY, 2004

Robbins, John
The Food Revolution: How Your Diet Can Help Save Your Life and the World
Red Wheel/Weiser, York Beach, ME, 2001

4 colon detoxification

The colon is the sewage system of the body. Neglected and abused, it becomes a cesspool. The cleaner your colon, the healthier you are going to be. Your greatest keys to health are fasting one day a week and having two bowel movements a day.

benefits of a cleansing program

- Dissolve and break up mucoid matter
- Rapidly expel mucoid matter from the system
- Cause no cramping
- Reduce gas in the stomach and intestines
- Kill any possible infection
- Heal any sore
- Purify the blood
- Stimulate and strengthen organs, especially the heart, liver, and eliminative organs
- Increase the secretions of the liver, pancreas, and stomach
- Strengthen, heal, and rebuild the peristaltic action as well as the entire digestive system
- Take away appetite
- Calm the nervous system and reduce possible pain
- Kill some worms
- Stop any hemorrhages

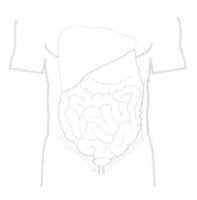

AUTOINTOXIFICATION

The process by which the body becomes poisoned from its own waste is called *autointoxification*. If your colon isn't clean and functioning properly, waste matter will not be eliminated. Instead, the toxic residue will be reabsorbed into your system and will cause numerous health problems, such as bad breath, body odor, putrid gas, digestive problems, acne, prostate problems, liver and gallbladder trouble, and chronic illness. Approximately 36 known poisons can exist in the colon, including indican, ammonia, cadaerin, and histidine.

Colon problems and the subject of elimination are not the most popular topics of conversation, yet millions of people are concerned. The news media constantly inform us of current statistics and narrate accounts of people who suffer from colon-related problems. Stop and think about the following information and how it could affect you.

laxatives. More than 40 million Americans spent $5 million on laxatives last year. This does not include the millions of dollars spent on bulking agents such as psyllium and Metamucil.

cancer. The second leading cause of death in the United States today is cancer, and 100,000 people die annually from colon cancer. According to the National Cancer Society, "Evidence in recent years suggests that most colon cancer is caused by environmental agents. Some scientists believe that a diet high in beef or low in fiber is the cause."

colitis, ileitis, diverticulitis, crohn's disease, irritable bowel syndrome (IBS). These conditions affect tens of millions of people, resulting in lost work time, disability, depression, and hospitalization; they are at the root of many common ailments.

colostomy. Thousands of people worldwide have colostomies every month, each procedure requiring the removal of a portion of the colon. The person must then eliminate solid waste through an opening in the side of the body into an attached pouch. This pouch is emptied and cleaned several times a day. Doctors who practice preventive medicine believe this drastic surgery can be prevented by a nutritional approach.

HISTORY OF COLON HYDROTHERAPY

Colon therapy is an ancient healing method used in many civilizations. The "Ebers Papyrus," an ancient Egyptian medical document, records the use of enemas as early as 1500 B.C.

Enemas were more common at one time in this country than they are today. General knowledge and use of this valuable health tool have decreased greatly in the past 50 years, but in our grandparents' and great-grandparents' time, the use of enemas was a widely accepted procedure for reversing the onset of illness.

With the development of sophisticated colonic irrigation machines and the increasing popularity of more natural health methods, colon hydrotherapy is currently making a comeback. It is estimated that there may be as many as 2,000 colon therapists presently practicing in the United States.

Colon therapists and researchers of degenerative diseases have shown that a significant percent of body weight consists of accumulated waste. Such waste builds up in the blood vessels, the lymphatic system, the joints, and in intra- and extracellular regions. The largest amount is found in the colon. Up to 50 pounds of fecal waste can become impacted in the colon over decades of unhealthy eating.

Some of this partially digested food in the small intestine and colon passes into the bloodstream and is deposited as waste throughout the system. If these wastes are calories, they can show up as obesity. Excess minerals show up as arthritis, excess protein leads to cancer, excess fat contributes to high cholesterol, and excess sugar leads to diabetes.

Colonic irrigation enables the impacted fecal matter to break down and be eliminated, along with particles of old mucus from the entire length of the colon. In some cases of cleansing, one or more forms of parasites, including tapeworms, may also be eliminated.

colonics. A colonic is an enema given by a professional colon hygienist or therapist using a colonic machine. The procedure is quite comfortable because the water circulates through the colon via a dual-flow tube and no pressure is built up as a result of water retention. Colonics are usually given in a series of 10 or more. In order to find a good colon hygienist, follow the recommendations of those you trust or, if possible, contact the International Association of Colonic Therapists (IACT).

revitalization program

The human mechanism is an elastic pipe system. Because much of the food we eat is never entirely digested and the resultant waste eliminated, our entire pipe system—and especially the digestive tract—slowly becomes constipated. This accumulated waste provides the foundation for every disease.

To loosen this waste and eliminate it intelligently and carefully is the goal of the revitalization program.

suggested reading
Jensen, Bernhard
Tissue Cleansing Through Bowel Management
Published by Bernard Jensen, D.C., Escondido, CA, 1981

---

causes of constipation
- Too little liquid
- Too little bulk
- Too little exercise
- Emotional tension
- Mechanical problems, such as a prolapsed colon
- Poor choice of foods
- Improper combination of foods
- Very hot or cold foods
- Weak muscle tone of the colon

constipating foods & drinks
- Cheese
- Fried foods
- Candies and sugar products
- White flour
- Salt and salted snack foods (potato chips, etc.)
- Beef
- Canned, burned, fermented, or processed food
- Pasteurized milk
- Wine with meals
- Carbonated drinks
- Coffee (has a drying effect on the colon)

If you are consuming these foods and drinks, your colon cannot possibly be healthy, even if you are having a bowel movement every day.

5 fasting

Fasting is a simple, quick, powerful way to cleanse the body and enhance healing from illness and disease. Fasting one day a week, every week of your life, can become your key to a healthier life.

Fasting

There's a hidden sweetness
in the stomach's emptiness.

We are lutes, no more, no less.
If the sound box is stuffed
full of anything, no music.

If the brain and the belly
are burning clean with fasting,
every moment a new song
comes out of the fire.

The fog clears, and a new
energy makes you run up the
steps in front of you.

Be emptier and cry like
reed instruments cry.
Emptier, write secrets with
the reed pen.

When you're full of food and drink,
Satan sits where your
spirit should, an ugly metal
statue in place of the Kaaba.

When you fast, good habits gather
like friends who want to help.

Fasting is Solomon's ring.
Don't give it to some illusion
and lose your power.

But even if you've lost all
will and control, they come
back when you fast,
like soldiers appearing out
of the ground, pennants
flying above them.

A table descends to your
tent, Jesus' table.
Expect to see it, when you
fast, this table spread with
other food better than the
broth of cabbages.

—Rumi

Fasting has been known for hundreds of years as a compensation or counterbalancing force against every disease. But why has it never come into general use in this country? Because it has not been used systematically, taking into account the condition of the patient. It is only in recent years that the medical profession is studying the broad-reaching reparative properties of the fast. Joel Fuhrman, M.D., (New Jersey) and Max Gerson, M.D., (Bonita, CA) are some of the pioneers.

The average person has not the slightest idea what the necessary eliminative process is, the time it requires, how the diet must be changed and how often, or what it means to cleanse the body of the terrible quantities of waste that accumulate in the process of living.

Disease can be understood as an effort by the body to eliminate accumulated waste, mucus, and toxins. Fasting assists nature in the most perfect and natural way, with ease rather than through disease. Remember: Accumulated wastes throughout your entire system are the source of every disease. Lowered vitality, imperfect health, lack of strength and endurance, and any other imbalances—all have their source in an unclean colon, especially a colon that has been inadequately cleaned since birth.

Many people are afraid of fasting. They believe it may be detrimental or possibly even dangerous to their health; they are also afraid of feeling deprived. Joel Fuhrman, M.D., has stated: "To fast is to abstain from food while one possesses adequate reserves to nourish vital tissues; to starve is to abstain from food after reserves have been exhausted so that vital tissues are sacrificed." Fasting is a simple, quick, powerful way to cleanse the body and to enhance healing from illness and disease.

During fasting no solid food at all is eaten, but liquids are consumed in large quantities. Liquids can include delicious raw fruit and vegetable juices, preferably fresh, since juices lose much of their valuable vitamins, minerals, trace elements, and enzymes within minutes of juicing. Vitamin-rich vegetable broths can also be utilized, as well as herb teas.

SOME BENEFITS OF FASTING

1. During a fast the body lives on itself; after three days, it burns and digests its own tissues, starting with those that are diseased, damaged, old, or dead.
2. The process of building new, healthy cells is speeded up.
3. The capacity of the lungs, liver, kidneys, and skin to process waste greatly increases, and masses of toxins are eliminated.
4. Digestive, assimilative, and protective organs are allowed to rest.
5. Vital physiological and mental functions are normalized, stabilized, and rejuvenated.

Detox and Revitalize: The Holistic Guide for Renewing Your Body, Mind, and Spirit

Fasting is beneficial as a general health measure. Many sources advise fasting regularly to keep the body clean. Fasting can also be of value when beginning to desensitize the body to certain foods or substances. You can see whether and how you overeat and assess your reliance on coffee, tea, cigarettes, alcohol, and certain foods such as refined sugar. Fasting may help you overcome those addictions.

Fasting can be done for one meal a day, for one day, or for many days at a time, or for as long as one week or several weeks.

PREPARATION FOR THE FAST

Eight days prior to the beginning of the fast, eat only fruit, raw and steamed vegetables, vegetable soups, fresh raw vegetable juices, some diluted fruit juices, herbal teas, olive oil, aloe vera juice, prune juice, and an herbal laxative tea daily.

supplements:

3 oz. prune juice in morning
1 cup laxative tea nightly
2 Tbsp. olive oil at bedtime
3 oz. aloe vera juice twice per day
Dry skin brushing: Five minutes first thing in the morning, then shower. Five minutes at bedtime, then shower. Use a natural vegetable fiber brush only. Be sure not to use any oils or lotions on your skin.

exercise:

Mini-trampoline exercises: Bounce on the rebounder at least 10 minutes per day.
Walk 20 minutes per day.
Take a detoxification bath each day.

detox drink—internal fiber cleanser

A fiber drink containing seeds ground into a powder, the Detox Drink, when mixed with water, absorbs 10 times its volume. As it expands, it acts as an internal brush, cleaning the entire alimentary canal, which is approximately 30 feet in length. This fiber drink should be an integral part of any fasting regime.

Detox drink

8 oz. water
2 oz. apple juice
1 Tbsp. intestinal fiber cleanser (see resource section)

Mix all ingredients, shake well, and drink fast.

FASTING: SEVEN-DAY "REVITALIZATION" PROGRAM

Have one of the following 12 drinks every hour or hour and a half. Use only distilled or purified water.

1. 2 capsules of enzymes and a glass of water
2. 1 Tbsp. chlorophyll and a glass of water
3. 1 cup of vegetable broth: Boil a few veggies and drink the broth only
4. *1st Detox Drink* of water, apple juice, and intestinal fiber cleanser (Fiber cleansers are available at all health food stores. They are often made of flax or psyllium.)
5. 1 pint vegetable juice (freshly made): carrot, celery, beets, cabbage
6. *2nd Detox Drink* of water, apple juice, and intestinal fiber cleanser
7. 1 cup of lemon water (1 fresh-squeezed lemon) and 1 capsule each of garlic, capsicum, and parsley
8. 1 cup energizing tea (yerba mate or green tea)
9. 1 cup blood-purifying tea (lapacho or Pau d'Arco)
10. 1 cup of tea for liver and kidneys (parsley and dandelion)
11. *3rd Detox Drink* of water, apple juice, and intestinal fiber cleanser, plus 20 drops of colloidal minerals followed with 3 capsules of acidophilus
12. 1 cup herbal laxative

For Best Results:

- 1 Tbsp. castor oil treatment the first day of the fast (mixed with 4 oz. prune or apple juice).
- Enema (or colema or colonic) each day.
- Retention enema every night (for instructions, see p. 19).
- Jump 10 minutes on the trampoline three times a day.
- Take a sauna or steam bath each day.
- Do skin brushing twice a day.
- Walk 20 minutes and take a detoxification bath each day.
- Forty-five minutes of yoga stretches, breathing, and relaxation each day will help the detoxification process.
- Repeat the seven-day revitalization program four times a year.

BREAKING THE FAST

The way you break your fast is very important! People have actually died breaking the fast the wrong way. A couple who visited We Care in 1990 did not take the information seriously and on Friday, after fasting all week, they went out to eat fried Chinese food. Their bodies were not able to handle the food, and we had to call the paramedics to pump their stomachs. So please pay attention!

However long you fast, remember that you have not digested any food while you have been fasting, and you must now train your body to digest again. If a runner is bedridden for a year, he cannot just get right up and run 20 miles. He must walk, then jog, then run. The longer you fast, the longer you must be careful coming off the fast. For every week of fasting, you must be careful for two or three days.

You should not eat potatoes, bananas, grains, toast, pasta, meats, or cheeses, even though your body may crave these foods in order to stop cleansing. Watery foods like raw or steamed vegetables are best.

Most important, you must have small meals, such as a serving of steamed vegetables, a bowl of soup, a piece of fruit, or a small salad. Be careful to chew your food well. You may have three meals, but it is better to have only two meals a day. That will also leave you time to drink enough fluid. Your body needs half of its pounds of body weight in ounces of liquid a day. For example, if you weigh 120 pounds, you need 60 ounces of liquid every day (certain medical conditions may require consultation with your medical doctor first). You may add more colonics or enemas after the fast.

We suggest the following home program and supplements in order to cleanse and rebuild your body all year long.

COMING OFF THE FAST

instructions

For the following three days:
- Eat very small meals.
- Eat only fresh vegetables (raw or steamed).
- Eat fresh fruit.

Breakfast

1 glass of fruit juice followed 15 minutes later by a piece of fruit

Lunch

1 glass of vegetable juice followed 15 minutes later by a vegetable salad

Dinner

1 glass of herbal tea followed 15 minutes later by a bowl of light vegetable soup

suggested supplements

Upon Rising

1 Detox Drink (Refer to the directions for this fiber drink on page 31.)
Fresh lemon juice in water every morning

Mid-morning
Chlorophyll

With Meals
Continue taking your enzymes for digestion.
Take your daily food supplement to support your nutritional needs.

At Bedtime
Natural herbal laxative when needed

upon completion of your cleanse, rebuild your intestinal flora

Benefits of Probiotics: (Beneficial Bacteria)

- Manufacture nutrients: Produce B complex vitamins, antioxidants, short-chain fatty acids, amino acids, and vitamin K (for bone building and heart health). The cells that line the colon are replaced completely every week, and this process requires a lot of energy; they don't receive nutrients from the bloodstream as most tissues do, however. Vitamins, minerals, and nutrients needed by this organ are all made by the probiotics that live along its walls.
- Boost immune system
- Slow cancer growth
- Fight infection
- Help prevent food allergies
- Fight yeast overgrowth
- Prevent and treat diarrhea and constipation
- Prevent and treat inflammatory bowel disease

Purchase a box of *Lactobacillus Bifidus* (we use Eugalan Topfer Forte, from Germany). Mix 3 scoops in a cup of warm water and drink daily—upon waking, with your lunch, and at bedtime—until the box is finished. Alternatively, purchase *lactobacillus bifidus* in capsule, tablet, or powder form at your local health food store and follow the directions on the label. Also purchase *acidophilus* and take 3 capsules, 3 times a day, together with the bifidus drink for 2 weeks, then take only 2 at night for maintenance.

Drink one glass of kefir each morning on an empty stomach. Kefir contains beneficial bacteria and does not feed yeast. Homemade kefir has more beneficial bacteria than yogurt, so you may want to make your own from soy or goat milk. Kefir has a laxative effect and also keeps the small and large intestines free from parasites. Kefir contains complete protein; many B vitamins, including B_{12}; and all the essential fatty acids. It is a natural antibiotic.

Kefir

1 quart milk (soy or goat)
5 grams Kefir Starter culture

Pour starter culture into a small glass. Pour 2 oz. of milk over the starter and stir until dissolved. Pour remaining milk into a glass container and add the dissolved mixture. Stir well. Pour all of the mixture into the kefir maker. Plug in for 10 hrs. Then refrigerate.

Uses:
Plain, or with fruit, or over a baked potato, or on a salad. Makes a good substitute for cream.

Yógourmet makes a good kefir starter kit. For more information on the benefits of kefir and making kefir, you can visit www.kefir.com.au <http://www.kefir.com.au/>.

Kefir Ice Cream

1 cup kefir
1 cup frozen strawberries
1/2 banana
1/2 tsp. vanilla extract

Mix all ingredients in a "Vita-Mix" and serve.

suggested reading

Mindell, Earl, PPH, Ph.D.
User's Guide to Probiotics
Basic Health Publications, North Bergen, NJ, 2004

Shahani, Khem M., Ph.D.
Cultivate Health from Within: Dr. Shahani's Guide to Probiotics
Vital Health Publishing, Danbury, CT, 2005

Fuhrman, Joel, M.D.
Fasting and Eating for Health
St. Martin's Press, New York, NY, 1998

6 maintenance program

Your maintenance program should be easy to follow.

five days per week, eat only organic:

- fresh salads
- vegetables—steamed, grilled,or sautéed
- vegetable soups
- whole pastas
- whole grains
- legumes
- seeds and nuts
- fresh fruits
- fresh juices and herb teas

If you are semivegetarian, occasionally add some grilled fish, breast of chicken (organic), and eggs (no antibiotics, no hormones)

One day per week, fast! One day per week, eat anything you want!

MAINTENANCE

Fast one day a week for four weeks.

The fourth week (or once a month), fast for three days in a row (at the full moon).

Every three months, fast for a complete week. During that week, you can do an enema in the morning and one at night.

one-day fast

Fasting lemonade

1 gallon of purified water
the juice of 5 lemons
5 tablespoons of maple syrup or 10 drops of liquid stevia extract

Mix water, lemon juice, and sweetener together. Drink 1 cup every hour. (Commercial lemonade will not work.)

For a Semifast

Add one simple meal a day, such as green salad, steamed vegetables, or fresh fruit.

parasites

Parasites are the cause of many diseases. It is a healthy practice to eat foods that are natural antiparasites, such as pumpkin seeds, garlic, and black walnuts. Avoid foods that may have parasites like pork, sushi, or any raw or semiraw meat.

As a preventive measure, do a parasite cleanse once or twice a year with natural herbs, such as Paracleanse from Nature Sunshine. Follow the instructions for 10 days. Stop the treatment for 10 days, then repeat for 10 days. Make sure to drink lots of fluids and eat light meals (vegetables and fruits only). Taking Paracleanse or another herbal parasite treatment can enhance your fast, but it is not necessary that you fast while taking it.

Liver flush

4 oz. aloe vera
2 cloves fresh garlic
1 fresh-squeezed lemon
3 Tbsp. olive oil
1 fresh-squeezed orange
dash of cayenne

Mix ingredients in the blender. Drink once a month, after your fasting day.

On a Full-moon Day

An alternative to the monthly liver flush is to fast on juices and teas for a full day. Take 30 drops of orthophosphoric acid three times a day (dissolves liver and gall stones). At bedtime: mix 3 oz. virgin olive oil and 3 oz. lemon juice; drink, and retire immediately. Next morning have an enema or a colonic.

for liver weakness

Eliminate oil or fat as much as possible, and eat absolutely no fried foods! Drink beet juice, eat beets (raw or steamed), steamed artichokes. Drink lemon juice daily, and use olive oil.

six-month colon rejuvenation program

Take daily:

- 1 glass of homemade kefir each morning, with added acidophilus
- 1 Detox Drink each morning
- 3 oz. aloe vera in a glass of juice (twice a day, between meals)
- chlorophyll (liquid, powder, or capsule) between meals
- 2 enzymes with each meal
- 2 aloe vera capsules, natural laxative when needed
- 3 acidophilus capsules at bedtime

Eat lots of fibrous foods (fruits, vegetables, seeds, nuts, whole grains, and legumes), and drink lots of liquids. Fast once a week, and take an enema, colema, or colonic therapy periodically.

Remember, 80 percent of hospital admissions are for lifestyle-related, preventable diseases. Some of these avoidable and reversible diseases are arteriosclerosis, coronary artery disease, arthritis, obesity, diabetes, hypoglycemia, hypertension, chronic pulmonary diseases, gastric ulcers, depression, and stress-related illness.

DAILY MAINTENANCE SUPPLEMENTS

To help the three most important functions of the body: digestion, assimilation, and elimination:

- Detox Drink—Intestinal fiber cleanser that helps remove debris from the intestinal tract. *Suggested:* take once daily for maintenance and twice daily while fasting (see p. 31).
- Enzymes—Break down food to help digestion (amylase to digest carbohydrates, protease for protein, lactase for lactose, lipase for fats, cellulase for cellulose). Take at the beginning of each meal.

- **Green energy food**—Any of the following or a mixture: chlorophyll, chlorella, spirulina, alfalfa, barley, and wheat grass. *Suggested:* take once or twice daily between meals.
- **Probiotics**—Reintroduce beneficial bacteria into the intestines (acidophilus, bifidum, and longum). *Suggested:* take once daily with kefir and twice daily for one month after fasting.
- **Colloidal minerals**—Aid vitamin absorption. Take the daily requirement once a day.
- **Natural herbal laxative**—Take only when needed. Try cascara sagrada or aloe vera. (See herbal reference section, pp. 126–131.)

Reach your goal of high energy and health by using these items regularly (whole super foods dehydrated into a powder).

- **Goat's whey**—Proteins and minerals from goat milk (can be used as coffee replacement in smoothies and other recipes).
- **Energy tea**—Yerba mate or decaffeinated Green Tea (can be used as coffee replacement).
- **Chlorophyll**—Is the blood of the plants, almost identical to human blood. It rebuilds your blood.
- **Rice bran solubles**—Rice bran solubles provide vitamins, minerals, amino acids and essential fatty acids, and antioxidants. We recommend a product called Life Solubles by Integris, available only from Integris distributors (see resources).
- **Lecithin**—Brain food and weight-loss helper, helps lower cholesterol.

other salts

Many doctors readily acknowledge that ordinary table salt, which is almost 100 percent sodium chloride, can produce harmful effects in the body. The common concern is the sodium/potassium imbalance.

Dr. Henry Gilbert, an early pioneer in this field, found that if ordinary table salt "had all the other salts of the body combined with it in correct physiological proportions, it would be a food; but when only one element is present, the mineral balance of the body is completely upset, and so the body is poisoned."

He further explained that ordinary salt interferes with the normal flow of all the fluids of the body and so tends to increase susceptibility to colds and other infectious ailments. It creates mineral imbalances and a relative deficiency of every other mineral constituent of the body. Then by displacing potassium in the cells, it causes a potassium deficiency.

Biochemist Jacques Loeb also affirmed that sodium chloride is poisonous to protoplasm unless combined with other essential elements.

In addition, Dr. C. Samuel West, a noted researcher on the lymphatic system, claims that ordinary table salt upsets the delicate mineral balance in and around the cells, thus interfering with the electrical function of the cell.

BioSalt: Biochemically Balanced

BioSalt is a triturated homeopathic compound preparation, biochemically balanced to correspond to the normal saline content of healthy human plasma, in the ratio the body uses it. Its active ingredients are: sodium chloride, potassium chloride, tricalcium phosphate, magnesium oxide, zinc oxide, potassium iodide, ferrous fumarate, copper gluconate, manganese sulphate, chromium picolinate, and trace minerals from sea salt.

Sea Salt

In considering sea salt as a possible alternative to ordinary table salt, researchers learned that sea salt contains too much magnesium and insufficient potassium, since humans, like other land animals, require more potassium than do sea creatures.

Salty Liquid Seasonings

Salty liquid seasonings made from soy, alfalfa, corn, or dulse, or a combination of these have no salt added, but they have a salty flavor. They also have no calories. They add great flavor to soups, salads, steamed veggies, noodles, rice, and sandwiches. I recommend We Care's My-Protein, Jensen's Quick Sip, Bragg's Liquid Aminos, or a high-quality, wheat-free tamari. You can also use a broth made from miso.

sweeteners

Stevia

A sweetener from a natural plant, stevia comes in both liquid and powder form. It has no calories. Much sweeter than sugar, it can be used for cooking and as a replacement for sugar and artificial sweetener. Good for diabetics.

Brown Rice Syrup
Pure Maple Syrup
Agave Nectar

vitamins and minerals

Vitamin E
Vitamin C
Vitamins A and D
Calcium and Magnesium—for healthy bones
Methylsulfonylmethane (MSM)—natural anti-inflammatory

7 enzymes, your fountain of youth

It is not what you eat but what you digest and assimilate that increases your energy and vitality. Enzymes help to break down food for proper assimilation of nutrients.

a healthy diet

Sixty-five percent raw foods (fresh juices, salads, nut milk, and fruit). Thirty-five percent cooked foods (steamed vegetables, grains, and legumes).

grains

Grains are seeds that need to be soaked overnight and cooked in the same water.

nuts and seeds

These must be soaked overnight for the enzymes to be released. The five most balanced nuts and seeds are almonds, sesame, pumpkin, sunflower, and flax. Some of the others are acid-forming and constipating.

legumes

Legumes must also be soaked overnight, but the water should be thrown away because it creates gas. Cook in fresh water.

energy

Sixty percent of our energy is spent trying to digest food. The more you feed your body easy-to-digest foods, the more energy you will have. Easy-to-digest foods include liquid meals, juices, fruits, and vegetables.

Enzymes are a part of every living cell. There are about 100,000 enzymes in every cell. Enzymes transform grape juice into wine, barley into beer, and apple juice into cider. They are essential for digestion because they transform the food you eat into the nutrients your body needs. An enzyme deficiency must be considered as a possible precursor to bodily imbalance and consequent disease symptoms.

Because enzymes are destroyed once they have completed their appointed task, you need a constant supply of these vital catalysts. Enzymes need to be supplemented in the diet just as you supplement minerals and vitamins.

Enzymes come from the foods you eat as well as from your own body. Good sources of enzymes include raw fresh vegetables and fruits, nuts and seeds (unroasted), fresh eggs (if you find a good source), and raw goat's milk. You can drink your enzymes too: Freshly squeezed raw vegetable juice has a very high enzyme content. You need all these enzymes to help your body digest food.

The biggest enemy of enzymes is heat. In any food or drink that has been heated over 118 degrees, the enzymes have been totally destroyed. When you eat cooked foods, your body overworks because it must produce twice as many digestive enzymes! Rejuvenate by fasting and by eating raw foods.

how to produce enzymatic power to digest your foods

1. **Relax.** You need to relax and have a clear mind when you eat. If you are tense, you cannot secrete the enzymes needed to digest your food properly. We tend to do the opposite—when we've just had an argument with a lover or friend, the first thing we do is go to the refrigerator.
2. **Chew your food well.** The more you chew, the less work your body has to do to break down food. For further discussion of this important point, see the next section on "Keeping Your Intestinal Tract Clean."
3. **Do not drink with your meals.** Doing so dilutes the digestive juices that break down the food. Drink one-half hour before your meal or two hours after your meal. Drink, in ounces, half of your body weight in pounds every day.
4. **Avoid hot or cold.** Don't drink your liquids too hot because they can burn the lining in your stomach where the enzymes are produced. Drinking very cold liquids puts the enzymes into a dormant stage.
5. **Eat only when your stomach is empty.** Wait four to five hours between solid meals and have liquid meals in between.

KEEPING YOUR INTESTINAL TRACT CLEAN

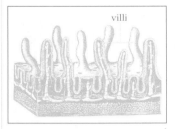

Everything you eat must be transformed into liquid. If the food is liquefied when it arrives at the small intestine, at this point the liquid transforms into gas. The gas passes through the walls of the intestinal tract and reaches the blood. The blood then undergoes a chemical change that allows it to carry the nutrients to every cell in the body.

The small intestine, which curls up around the belly, is about 22 feet long. In the cross-section you can see that its surface is corrugated rather than flat. Each curl contains hundreds of little fingers called villi. Within the villi are microscopic holes through which the nutrients pass to reach the bloodstream. But if these microscopic holes are plugged up, how can the nutrients pass through them? The cleaner the intestinal tract, the more nutrients can be delivered to your tissues and cells, and the healthier and more energetic you are going to be.

So what can plug up the villi? If you throw a gallon of fat in your sink, the sink immediately becomes plugged up. Remember this when you eat fatty foods. Animal fat (all meats), dairy products full of animal fat, and fried foods clog the villi. White flour and white rice products do the same. Since these foods work against us, we need to avoid them.

What foods can help clean up this mess? Watery foods that pass easily through the villi. So drink more water, juices, herbal teas, and powdered (dehydrated) foods that you dissolve and drink. Prepare more smoothies in the blender and eat more fruits and vegetables because they are 70 percent water. That is all you need to know about nutrition: Avoid foods that clog the villi—meats, dairy products, fried foods, and white flour products—and enjoy lots of liquid nutrients and fruits and vegetables.

intestinal detox

Now, what can you do to clean up the mess created from years of eating the wrong way? One major reason for creating this manual is to learn how to clean up all the debris in a safe and intelligent way.

This is how it is done: Every hour on the hour, you drink water, water and lemon, herbal teas, vegetable juices, and chlorophyll. This soaks the intestinal tract.

Next, you take a Detox Drink, which functions as a "Roto Rooter" or intestinal brush (see p. 31). It contains fiber in powdered form (from organic flax seed, apple pectin, oat bran, or psyllium). When you mix it with water, it absorbs 10 times its volume and acts like a brush, brushing the 30 feet of piping from the mouth to the anus.

Once the Detox Drink has moved the debris to the large intestine (which is four to five feet long), natural laxatives (aloe vera juice, prune juice, herbal laxatives, olive or castor oil) and colon hydrotherapy help to move all the unwanted "old stuff" out of your body. Breaking down the old food and carrying it out of the body may take days, and sometimes weeks, of repeating the same process.

To keep your system in good health, you need to cleanse periodically on a regular basis. Fasting is a way of life. Eating well is a way of life. You clean up your system with juices, teas, fruits, and vegetables, because the cleaner your body, the more energy you enjoy. We suggest continuing to take the Detox Drink on a daily basis even when you are not fasting, because this internal brushing helps you to stay clean. Eating fiber regularly is also a good healthy habit: fruits, vegetables, seeds and nuts, whole grains, and legumes. Avoid nonfiber foods such as meat, dairy products, eggs, white flour, and white sugar.

why are enzymes so important?

Each of us is born with a pool of enzymes. These enzymes are designed to create brand new cells. The size of this enzyme pool is directly related to the health of your parents. If you come from healthy parents, your enzyme bank will most likely be large. If your parents had frail health, your enzyme bank may be deficient. If you were breast-fed, your pool of enzymes increased because mother's milk contains a tremendous number of enzymes. On the other hand, if you were fed formula or pasteurized milk, or any man-made product without enzymes, you began to rob your enzyme bank from day one of your life.

Every time you eat a cooked meal, a meal with no enzymes, your body robs enzymes from your enzyme bank to digest the cooked food. Enzymes that were originally designed to create new cells are withdrawn from the enzyme bank and used for digestion. In this way, you may rob your enzyme bank until your account is almost exhausted.

So what can you do to remedy this situation? You can use the power of fasting. The power of fasting lies in its rejuvenating power. When you fast, you stop robbing your enzyme bank and begin to build it up again. Because you are not digesting any food, you do not need any enzymes for digestion. At the same time, you drink enzymes all day long—first, two capsules on an empty stomach, then fresh juices, lemonade, and the chlorophyll drink.

Where do the enzymes go? They go to rebuild your liver, your kidneys, your heart—every cell, tissue, and organ of your body. They go to rebuild your enzyme bank. Fasting rejuvenates every cell of your body. This is why it is so beneficial to incorporate one day of fasting, or semifasting, into your lifestyle on a weekly basis. It is the most important tool you have for getting stronger and healthier!

Again, why are enzymes so important? Because enzymes and minerals are needed for the creation of new cells. Your body produces 2.5 billion red blood cells per second. Without enzymes and minerals, how can new cells be produced? When your enzyme bank is used up, you die. This is why a diet rich in enzymes, full of fresh organic fruits and vegetables, is so important.

When I say "fresh," I mean produce full of life force, freshly picked from the fields or trees, food that travels directly from the growing plant to your mouth. "Fresh" does not mean packaged, because packaged food in any form is no longer vital. It is not poisonous, but it does not contain the life force your body needs to stay well. Where are the minerals? In fresh organic plant life. And where does the plant get the minerals? From the soil. You can eat spinach until the day you die, but if iron, calcium, and other minerals are missing from the soil in which the seed is planted, there will be no minerals in the spinach, no matter how big and showy the plant may look because of added fertilizers. So make an effort to eat more fresh organic produce, the vital source of minerals and enzymes. And add a colloidal mineral supplement to your diet.

The following sections are adapted, with permission, from *If The Buddha Came to Dinner* by Hale Sofia Schatz.

EATING VS. FEEDING

In my experience, the discipline of nourishing your body can be an amazingly effective vehicle for spiritual development and transformation. How can feeding yourself be a spiritual practice? If food seems more mundane than yoga or meditation or prayer, that's because it is. Food is one of our primary human needs. Many times a day, every day, you put some kind of food in your mouth. When you consume food without much thought beyond its taste, I call it *eating*. You know what eating looks like: It's the compulsive reaching into the bag of potato chips; eating when you're full because food is just there; grabbing a quick bite for lunch between meetings; indulging your taste buds while ignoring how your body feels.

When you make deliberate food choices based on your need for a diet rich in enzymes—foods that support physical energy, mental clarity, creativity, and focus—I call this *feeding oneself*. I use these terms to emphasize the difference between mindless consumption and purposeful, conscious fueling. The term feeding oneself also shows how transformational nourishment requires two components: the part of yourself that does the nourishing (*feeding*) and the part that receives it (*oneself*). When you feed yourself, you are aware of and responsive to your particular needs for nourishment in the present moment.

LEARNING TO RECEIVE

When you are nourished, you are fulfilled. You feel a pervasive sense of well-being. And it is enough. Yet how often do you really let yourself feel that something is enough? Nourishment requires both giving and receiving. The giving part of nourishment can be easy—making a fresh salad, homemade soup, grilled vegetables. But receiving may not be so easy. I know loving people who give generously to their families and friends and yet have a very difficult time receiving from others, including themselves.

You cannot be nourished if you don't allow yourself to receive. To receive nourishment, you need to be open—but not just to take in food. Transformational nourishment means that your body, heart, mind, and spirit are open and willing to take in the nourishment that is offered to you from the universe. To do this, you need to know from the bottom of your heart that you are valuable and worthy to receive.

suggested reading
Schatz, Hale Sofia
If The Buddha Came to Dinner
Hyperion, New York, 2004

8 easy changes for a healthier life

Easy does it! Do not get overwhelmed.

Just take it one step at a time.

avoid nonfoods:

Cold cuts

Pork and red meat

White flour

White sugar

Fried foods, fat

Salt

Dairy products

Processed foods

Coffee

Sodas

grains

1st choice—Whole grains
soaked and cooked slowly

2nd choice—Flourless bread
(from sprouted grains)

3rd choice—Whole-grain
breads and pasta (artichoke,
quinoa, whole millet, brown
rice, etc.)

4th choice—no choice—
White flour (bread, pasta, and
pastries)

Best grains: millet and
quinoa

1. **Eggs.** Commercial chickens and eggs are full of hormones that stimulate faster reproduction. These hormones affect your own hormonal system. Switch to organic, free-range eggs.

2. **Meat.** If you still eat meat, fish, or chicken, eat small amounts and buy only organic or free-range products from the health food store. You can mix these meats with steamed vegetables, salads, or soups. Do not mix them with bread, pasta, grain, or baked potato. The best way to cook the meats is under the broiler or on the grill, letting the fat drip away.
   - Avoid packaged meats such as bologna, salami, ham, sausages, hot dogs, and turkey (compressed meats with preservatives, additives, and the like).
   - Pork and ham have the highest fat content. These animals often carry parasites.
   - Beef has a high fat content, and it is in the fat that chemicals accumulate.
   - Fish contain all the poisons that we are throwing in the ocean. Industrial companies are dumping large quantities of mercury, and whole colonies of fish are dying.

3. **Flour.** The center of the grain is white starch or glue; the outside brown shell contains all the oils and nutrients. White flour and white rice are products of a chemical process that removes the outside shell—and all the nutrients—leaving just the starchy center of the grain. Commercially, this process is more profitable than leaving the grain whole, because whole grains need to be refrigerated and spoil in a short time. By using white, refined products, producers avoid the cost of using refrigerated trucks for transport and eliminate spoilage.

   Our bodies, however, are not designed to digest white flour; to handle it, the body must take from its own reserve of minerals stored in the bones. (The bones are the storehouse of vitamins and minerals.) Please avoid all white flour products.

4. **Whole Grains.** Include only whole grains in your diet. Whole grains can be defined as kernels that occur the way they originated from nature. Whole grains can be left intact, ground, cracked, or flaked. Examples of devitalized or processed grains are enriched, bleached, or unbleached flour, and white rice. Remember that whole grains must be soaked overnight. Soaking converts the starch at the center of the grain into a little leaf composed of protein. Switch to whole grains.

5. **Sugar.** Sugar changes the composition of the mineral content of your blood. It especially affects calcium, sodium, and potassium. Eliminate all white sugar from your diet. Reduce other sugars as well: dextrose, maltose, fructose, corn syrup, brown sugar, and honey. They all have the same effect on your body. Switch to brown rice bran syrup, maple syrup, and stevia. Limit the intake of fresh fruits to one or two a day. Drink little or no fruit juice (one glass of fruit juice equals six to eight pieces of fruit).

6. **Oil.** A very important nutrient, eating the *right oils* improves energy level, athletic performance, fat loss, cardiovascular health, immune function, and longevity. You need no more than two tablespoons per day to lubricate the joints in the body. Good oil is raw, cold-pressed or cold-spelled. If this is not indicated on the label, the oil is *not* a good one. Good oils include virgin olive oil and cold-pressed flaxseed oil. Try Omega Essential Balance™. Other good cold-pressed oils are avocado, almond, sesame oil, and hemp oil. Hemp oil has all of the essential fatty acids in the perfect ratio.

    Eliminate anything that is hydrogenated or pasteurized, such as margarine, Crisco™, olestra, and canola oil.

    Do not cook with oil. Cooked oils and fats, as well as oils pressed under heat, change in molecular structure, becoming a solid molecule that your body cannot use for lubrication. These molecules stay in the veins and arteries, causing cholesterol buildup, hardening of the arteries, arteriosclerosis, and heart disease.

    Cook with water and serve the oil at the table. Keep oil refrigerated, and buy it in small amounts so it does not spoil.

    For grilled or sautéed vegetables only, use a small amount of olive oil or virgin coconut oil.

7. **Dairy Products.** These are mucus-forming, and also cause constipation. They contain fat, as well as many chemicals and pesticides. Use small amounts of unpasteurized goat milk and goat cheese, organic sheep milk and sheep cheese, or soy cheese. Substitute nut milk for cow's milk; nut butter for butter; soy cheese for cheese; and occasionally use goat or sheep cheese.

8. **Protein.** We need protein in the small amounts found in vegetables, grains, legumes, sprouts, and seeds. Most vegetable protein is an incomplete protein, which means it does not contain all the essential amino acids. Consequently, you must

avoid sugar:
Replace it with stevia (no calories) and occasionally maple syrup, brown rice syrup, or agave

avoid artificial sweeteners

eliminate:
Hydrogenated oils and transfat (margarine)
Olestra
Canola oil

"The Center for Science in the Public Interest (CSPI) today forwarded to the Food and Drug Administration (FDA) more than 200 new complaints of adverse reactions from consumers who had eaten snack foods containing the indigestible fat substitute olestra. With close to 20,000 reports forwarded to the agency from both CSPI and olestra developer Procter & Gamble, the FDA has logged more complaints about olestra than it has about all other food additives in history combined."
(4/16/02 CSPI press release)

learn to eat a wide variety of foods. Nutritious foods high in protein include avocados, nuts, seeds, sprouts, grains, legumes, and organic soy beans.

9. **Fruit.** Eat fruit alone. Fruit is a healthful snack, and eating one to two pieces of fruit per day is desirable. You can have fruit one-half hour before your meals or two hours after your meals. You can eat more strawberries, berries, and cantaloupe melons because they are very low in sugar.

NUTRITIONAL PROGRAM

Daily nutrition should include:
- 1 pint of fresh vegetable juice
- 1 glass of lemon water (1 freshly squeezed lemon)
- chlorophyll (liquid or powder)
- 1 large bowl of fresh green salad, including sprouts
- 1 or 2 pieces of fruit
- 2 cups of herb tea
- 1 cup of prepared goat's whey or miso
- 1 cup of homemade kefir from goat's milk
- 1 portion of nut milk
- 2 Tbsp. cold-pressed oil
- other foods to alternate: steamed vegetables, vegetable soups, grains, legumes, whole pasta, and organic soybeans (Edamame)

average day's diet

Upon Rising

A glass of water
30 minutes later, herbal tea and the Detox Drink (see p. 31)
30 minutes later, juice of a fresh lemon in a glass of water

Breakfast

- Smoothie: nut milk and fruit, (see pp. 74–75) (you may add 1 Tbsp. chlorophyll or 1 Tbsp. goat's whey, rice solubles, or lecithin)
- Kefir and a piece of fruit in the blender (see p. 80)
- Fresh vegetable juice (carrot, celery, beet, cabbage) (see pp. 78–79 for juicing recipes)

---

examples of healthy food combinations:

- Grains plus nuts and seeds
- Grains and legumes
- Avocado and sprouts
- Salads with sprouts and seeds
- Rice and beans with a salad
- Steamed vegetables with rice and nuts
- Baked potato, nut milk, and a salad
- Fruit and nut milk or kefir
- Soft-boiled, fertile eggs from free-range chickens could be a good source of protein during your transition diet.

Mid-morning

Energy Tea—yerba mate tea or decaffeinated organic green tea

Lunch

An enzyme, one multiple-vitamin, and one mineral tablet before lunch
Fresh green vegetable salad with sprouts and nut milk
(You may add baked potato, bowl of brown rice, or slice of flourless bread.)

2½ Hours After Lunch

Water, herb tea, or lapacho tea

Mid-afternoon

1 Tbsp. chlorophyll

Early Dinner

2 enzyme tablets before dinner
Choose two or three of the following:
- Salad, such as the Avocado Salad or Gourmet Cold Salad (recipes found on pp. 88–89)
- Steamed vegetables
- Bowl of soup, such as Susana's Super Soup (recipe, pp. 98–99)
- Noodles or whole grain or flourless bread
- Legumes and grains
- Avocado and sprouts (sandwich or salad)
- Organic steamed soybeans

Evening

1 cup of prepared goat's whey (coffee replacement) (recipe, pp. 80)

Bedtime

2 acidophilus capsules every night for maintenance

foods to avoid

- Dairy products such as milk, cheese, butter, etc.
- Refined carbohydrates such as sugar, white flour, white rice, pastries, cake, and breads
- Tea
- Coffee
- Chocolate
- Carbonated drinks
- Alcohol
- Tap water
- Dried fruit (use very little, and soak it)
- Vinegar (use lemon instead)
- Pork, red meats, shellfish, dark poultry, rabbits, organ meats
- Roasted and salted seeds and nuts (eat only raw or nut milk)
- Fried foods
- Fruit juices (very little—diluted only)
- Canned foods
- Cold cuts and prepared meats such as salami, bologna, ham, and hot dogs

If you go to www.theorganicpages.com then click on "Organic Ingredients," you can find organic food retailers by country and regions within those countries. A great resource for finding organic products quickly wherever you are. You can also find restaurants that serve organic food on this site.

GUIDE TO SHOPPING

shopping list

Buy organically grown food at your local health food stores. Many larger grocery chains now also stock organic produce. If there are no health food stores in your area, check out these internet sources for organic produce:

- Trader Joe's (50% organic), www.traderjoes.com
- Wild Oats, www.wildoats.com
- Whole Food Stores, www.wholefoods.com
- Vegetarian Source Online, www.vegsource.com
- Diamond Organics, www.diamondorganics.com

You can also contact your state's organic trade association for information on where to find organic products.

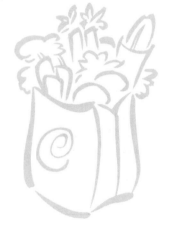

whole grains
Millet
Quinoa
Brown rice
Basmati brown rice
Wild rice
Steel-cut oats
Wheat kernels
Cracked wheat
Rye
Corn
Buckwheat
Spelt
Kamut

Buy whole grains, (brands like Arrowhead Mills, Harvest Quinoa, Lundburg, Now Foods, etc.) and healthful packaged hot and cold cereals and granola from organically grown, sugar- and salt-free whole grains (brands like Arrowhead Mills, Health Valley, Little Stream Bakery, Bread Shop, Familia, Very Pure, Life Stream, Nature's Path).

pasta and noodles made from:
Artichoke and semolina
Quinoa and semolina
Whole wheat
Whole durham flour
Corn
Oats

For sprouting instructions, visit www.sproutpeople.com

Rice
Spelt
Kamut
(Brands: De Boles, El Molino, Ancient Harvest Quinoa, Annie Chun's, Tinkyada) Avoid white, enriched, bleached, and unbleached flour.

breads, pastries, and crackers
Best are those made from sprouted or whole grains like wheat, rye, and mixed grains (100% flourless).
Whole wheat pita bread
Blue corn tortillas
Chapatis (made from lentil and rice flour)
(Brands: Oasis, Food for Life, Essene, Garden of Eden, French Meadow, Rudolph's, Nature's Path, Little Stream)
Avoid white, enriched, bleached, and unbleached flour.

oils (Note: Always add to foods at serving time, not for cooking)
Total: A maximum of 2 Tbsp. per day of any one of the following:
Flax seed oil
Hemp oil
Virgin olive oil
Cold-pressed almond, avocado, sesame, and sunflower
(Brands—not for cooking: Omega, Spectrum, Udo, Manitova Harvest, Now Foods)

nut butters
Almond butter
Sesame tahini butter
Cashew butter
Sunflower butter
Peanut butter (occasionally)
Avoid margarine, vegetable shortening, and animal fats.

seeds and nuts for nut milk (raw and unsalted)
Almonds
Hemp seeds
Flax seeds
Sesame seeds
Sunflower seeds
Pumpkin seeds
Cashews

recommended oils— always look for cold-pressed, organic oils
- Virgin olive oil
- Flax seed oil
- Hemp oil
- Virgin coconut oil (for cooking)

oils to avoid:
- Hydrogenated and transfat
- Olestra
- Canola
- Vegetable shortening
- Animal fat

coffee:

Highly acid-forming, should be avoided

substitute:

Yerba mate
Prepared goat's whey
Grain coffee substitute like Teecino, Celestial Seasonings Roastaroma, Pero Instant

sweeteners

- Stevia
- Rice bran syrup

salt

Use: BioSalt; sea salt; salty liquid seasoning like Jensen's Quick Sip, Bragg's Liquid Aminos, We Care's My-Protein, or a wheat-free tamari

avoid table salt

vinegar

Organic, unpasteurized apple-cider vinegar; other vinegars are acid-forming.

legumes

Beans (adzuki, pinto, black, kidney, moong, etc.)
Lentils
Garbanzo beans (also called chick peas)
Fresh or frozen Edamame (soy beans)
Green peas

beverages

Soy milk
Rice milk
Almond milk
Amasake
Coffee substitute, such as yerba mate, decaffeinated green tea, and goat's whey
Herbal teas
Purified water
Water and lemon

sweeteners

Cinnamon powder
Rice bran syrup (fructose-free)
Stevia (noncaloric, made from the chrysanthemum flower, good for diabetics and hypoglycemics) (Brands: Now Foods, Wisdom of the Ancients)

occasionally:
Maple syrup
Date crystals
Barley malt syrup
Honey
Agave

seasonings

BioSalt (salt substitute) or sea salt
Cayenne (pepper substitute)
Kelp
Fresh and dried herbs
Fresh lemon juice
Vinegar (unfiltered and unpasteurized, from apple cider)
Salty liquid seasoning (We Care's My-Protein, Jensen's Quick Sip, Bragg's Liquid Aminos, or high-quality, wheat-free tamari)
Carob (chocolate substitute) high in calcium and fiber
Cinnamon
Nutmeg

Natural vanilla extract

Agar-agar: tasteless, noncaloric vegetable gelatin from seaweed.

Arrowroot (to thicken sauces and soups); replacement for cornstarch.

Miso paste: barley and rice miso (for soups); rich in B complex. Buy unpasteurized. Avoid boiling.

Nutritional yeast: good cheese flavor for salads and soups; full of B complex. (Do not substitute brewer's yeast. KAL brand is good.)

protein

Edamame: organic soybeans.

Tempeh: like tofu, low in fat and calories and rich in nutrients. Made from soybeans.

sea vegetables (iodine and minerals)

Dulse

Wakame

Nori

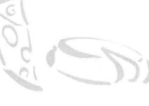

cheeses

Soy cheese

Goat cheese

Rice cheese

Seed cheese

eggs

Eat only organic, free-range eggs, with no antibiotics or hormones, purchased from your health food store.

It turns out that eggs are not such a bad food after all! The white of the egg is the protein. Two eggs will give you about 14 grams of protein. The yolk is mostly lecithin. Lecithin is food for the brain and nervous system; it helps digest fat, and so helps you lose weight and reduce cholesterol. If you cook the yolk, however, you destroy the lecithin, and cholesterol is created in the process of digesting the cooked yolk. So eat only "good" eggs and prepare them soft boiled, soft poached, sunny side up (but not fried), or eat them raw in your smoothie, your soup, or your noodles.

To avoid the risk of salmonella, soak the eggs in 1 gallon of water plus 1 Tbsp. of bleach for 10 minutes, then transfer them to the refrigerator.

candida diet:

Almost restricted to green leafy vegetables and grains like millet and quinoa

- No wheat
- No sugar
- No fruit juices
- Just one piece of fruit a day
- No dairy products, vinegar, soy sauce, sweets of any kind
- Increase your intake of acidophilus
- Keep cleansing the body
- No fermented foods
- No alcohol

note:

For more information on the Candida diet, read *Cultivate Health from Within: Dr. Shahani's Guide to Probiotics* by Khem Shahani, Ph.D. (Vital Health Publishing)

further suggestions

Condiments

BioSalt or sea salt, kelp, garlic, oregano, veggie salt, cayenne pepper, lemon, onion powder, basil

Juices

Fresh vegetable (15 minutes before your meals)

Herb Teas

Yerba mate, lapacho, decaffeinated organic green tea

breakfast ideas

1. Piece of fruit, melons (alone)
2. 1 oz. kefir or yogurt, 2 tsp. ground flax seed, stevia or agave to sweeten, fruit (optional: add 1 oz. Thai-Go liquid antioxidant.).
3. Smoothies: breakfast drink (mix in blender). Choose one:
    - Orange, lemon juice, apple, ground pumpkin seeds, carrot, beet
    - Raisins, coconut, banana, papaya, water
    - Apple, banana, orange, water, raisins, almonds
    - Avocado, cashews, banana, coconut, water

    To improve flavor, add: vanilla extract or carob powder.
    To improve nutrition, add: 1 Tbsp. chlorophyll, 1 Tbsp. goat's whey, 1 Tbsp. lecithin, 1 Tbsp. rice bran solubles.
4. Whole grain cereal, cooked, and served with nut milk. Choose one:
    - Millet
    - Quinoa
    - Oat
    - Rye
    - Seven grain
5. Fresh fruit (then wait 20 minutes), uncooked cereal (muesli) or cooked grain
6. Poached or soft-boiled eggs, sprouted grain bread, nut butter (raw sesame tahini or almond)

lunch or dinner ideas

1. Raw fruit salad (eat melons alone) plus goat kefir or yogurt or nut milk
2. Large vegetable salad (celery, spinach, cucumber, carrots, bell pepper, radishes, alfalfa sprouts or sunflower seeds, etc.) plus sprouted-grain bread or crackers, brown rice, ground seeds, soup or broth

3. Homemade vegetable soup plus small salad, baked potato, crackers or sprouted-grain bread, sesame butter
4. Steamed vegetables plus sprouted-grain bread or crackers, small salad, brown rice
5. Avocado and alfalfa sandwich on sprouted-grain bread, tomatoes, miso or raw sesame tahini, and an apple
6. Fish, baked or broiled, plus cooked vegetables, small salad
7. Brown rice and beans (or any other legume or grain) plus small salad, cup of soup, corn tortilla
8. Soup plus sprouted-grain bread, nut butter. Types of soup: vegetable, lentil, broccoli, miso broth, miso and mixed vegetable
9. Fertile eggs, goat and sheep cheeses, and fish may be eaten occasionally.

STAYING ON A HEALTHY DIET

To be able to stay on a healthful diet composed of lots of fresh organic vegetables and fruits with some grains, legumes, seeds, and nuts, your body must be maintained—kept "clean." If your body stays clean, you will not crave meats, fried foods, sugar, and other processed foods.

The practice of a one-day fast every week, and a one-week cleansing every three months is your best tool for accomplishing this.

Get your kitchen organized! Throw out all white flour, sugar, and canned food. Read labels. Do your shopping once a week, washing, drying, and packaging all your fresh vegetables and fruits. Prepare several dressings all at once to season your salads, steamed vegetables, noodles, grains, and so on. Cook extra rice, beans, lentils, and tomato sauce, and freeze an extra portion for *instant meals*. Drink fresh vegetable juice and lemon juice daily! Eat lots of salads and sprouts.

Create your own support group! Invite a couple of "health advocate" friends to a potluck to discuss, learn, and promote healthful living.

Buy books, magazines, cassettes, and videos containing health and environmental information to share. Support organizations dedicated to health research and enlightenment. Be an example!

And, remember: Movement is life! Breathing exercises, walks, yoga, and trampoline exercise should be incorporated into your daily routine for a healthier life.

suggested reading
Robbins, John
Diet for a New America
H. J. Kramer, Tiburon, CA, 1987

PUTTING IT ALL TOGETHER

1. Fast one day per week (drink hourly) or semifast (add only one simple meal, such as:
   - Green salad
   - Steamed vegetables
   - Vegetable soup
   - Fruit plate

2. Drink lots of fluids daily (every $1\frac{1}{2}$ hours)
   - Purified water
   - Water and lemon
   - Vegetable juice
   - Small fruit juice
   - Prepared goat's whey (p. 80)
   - Chlorophyll
   - Smoothies
   - Vegetable soup

3. Have two to three bowel movements daily.
   Take the Detox Drink daily, and drink lots of water.
   Take natural laxatives as needed. Alternate:
   - Kefir
   - Prune juice
   - Aloe vera juice
   - Aloe Vera capsules
   - Magnesium
   - Cascara sagrada
   - Olive oil
   - Castor oil

4. On a full-moon day (repeat every month):
   Fast, have an enema or colonic. Do a liver flush. Fast all day, have 30 drops of orthophosphoric acid three times a day. At bedtime, drink 3 oz. of fresh-squeezed lemon juice and 3 oz. of olive oil. Next morning, have an enema or colonic.

5. Eat lots of vegetables and fresh fruits:
   raw salads; steamed, grilled, sautéed vegetables; soups.

6. Eat only whole grains, legumes, seeds, and nuts.

7. Avoid nonfoods:
   - Cold cuts
   - Hot dogs
   - Pork

Dairy products
Fried foods
White flour
White sugar
Canned food
Coffee
Sodas

8. Learn to switch:
   - from milk to: nut milk, soy milk, rice milk
   - from cheese to: small amount of goat cheese, soy cheese, and rice cheese
   - from white flour bread to: organic, whole grain, or sprouted-grain breads
   - from white pasta to: whole durham, quinoa, spelt, Jerusalem artichoke, kamut, corn, rice
   - from oil to: virgin olive oil, Omega Essential Balance oil, flax oil, hemp oil
   - from margarine and butter to: nut butter (almond and sesame)
   - from regular ketchup to: sugar-free organic ketchup
   - from regular mustard to: sugar-free organic mustard
   - from coffee to: grain coffee, goat's whey, yerba mate
   - from white sugar to: stevia, rice bran syrup, honey, maple syrup, agave
   - from canned vegetables to: fresh and frozen vegetables

9. To help digestion, eat only two solid meals. Eat early during day hours. Take 2 capsules of enzymes before meals.

10. Get organized! Shop once a week. Wash, dry, and pack every vegetable. Prepare three dressings, enough for the week. Cook extra lentils, quinoa, rice, beans, soups, and so on.

11. When going out to eat, choose only healthy restaurants, order à la carte, specify a dressing of lemon and olive oil.

12. Exercise daily: walks, yoga, and trampoline.

When making health changes: Do not get overwhelmed.
   - Make a *few* changes at a time.
   - You do not have to be perfect, just *better*.
   - *Any* improvement is an improvement.

THE VEGETARIAN DECISION

1. Sixty percent of the energy we use each day is used for digestion. Fruits and vegetables, which consist of 70 percent water, require a lot less energy to digest than meats. Your body is like a machine and works under the same principles as any machine: The more work you give it to do, the more wear and tear on its parts, and the shorter its life span. If you have a brand new car and drive it 100,000 miles this year, next year you may need to buy a new car. So give your body a break with easy-to-digest foods like fruits and veggies. You will have more energy.

2. Animal fats (from all meats), dairy products from cows (which contain lots of animal fat), and fried foods contribute to many of the diseases and unhealthy conditions we suffer from today, such as arteriosclerosis, heart disease, high cholesterol, cancer, and obesity.

3. When you consume animal food like beef or poultry, you ingest all the chemicals that were fed to the animals: antibiotics, hormones, and pesticides.

4. High consumption of red and processed meat over a long period of time is associated with an increased risk for a certain type of colon cancer, according to a study in the January 12 issue of the *Journal of the American Medical Association*.

5. If you become vegetarian (or almost vegetarian), you will help balance the ecology on the planet. Today hundreds of acres of forest are being cut down to provide grazing land for cattle. We need those trees. They produce the oxygen we need to breathe, and they take in and use the carbonic acid we exhale.

6. Today we do not breed animals with the care and respect they deserve. We treat them like objects in factories designed for mass production. We will pay a high price for abusing them.

suggested reading

Robbins, John
Diet For a New America
H. J. Kramer, Tiburon, CA, 1998

Lyman, Howard
Mad Cowboy: Plain Truth From the Cattle Rancher
Who Won't Eat Meat
Simon & Schuster, New York, NY, 1998

"Susana will turn your life around with her nutritional guides—which I have happily followed for years."   —Barbara Rush, Actress

"No choice I have ever made has had a more beneficial impact on my quality of life than going vegan. I have been vegan for six years now and I still continue to experience more and more changes for the better, in every aspect of my life. The most obvious changes are physical—I have lost a lot of weight, I have an incredible amount of energy, and every part of me feels healthier and stronger than ever before. My skin is smoother, my eyes clearer, and my nails stronger.

"Going vegan has also brought me emotional and spiritual strength and peace. I am proud to be a woman who has made this choice and stands behind it. My choice brings me hope, pride, and a sense of accomplishment, for I now see that it is possible to effect change in the world, one person at a time. Living a vegetarian lifestyle, free of reliance on the suffering of living creatures, has an impact on every aspect of the world around us. I truly believe that by living this way we can heal the planet and make a more peaceful world. Food is our most basic need and that makes it our most powerful tool."   —Alicia Silverstone

"I was born and raised in Argentina, where my father was a cattle rancher, and for many years I ate meat three times a day. During my school years I suffered frequently from flus, colds, coughs, headaches, fevers, and constipation. About 25 years ago, I realized there was a direct connection between my diet and my health, and I became a vegetarian. Now I live on a diet of mostly organic fresh fruits and vegetables with a little rice, beans, whole pasta, lentils, and split peas, and occasionally, good eggs and goat or soy cheese. I fast and have a colonic and a massage regularly one day every week. I drink lots of fresh juices, herbal teas, and water with lemon. I feel strong and healthy.

"I opened the We Care center 17 years ago and have not missed a day of work yet. I do not take any medications or prescription drugs nor do I have pain anywhere in my body. I do yoga seven days a week and go out dancing four or five nights a week. I walk, soak in the hot detox bath, brush my skin, and take saunas regularly. I meditate and try to apply in my life the spiritual practices I have learned from all the great teachers I have met on my path. My vitality, strength, mental and emotional health are better than ever. Becoming a vegetarian has been a good change for me."   —Susana L. Belen

"Vegetarians have the best diet (and) the lowest rate of coronary heart disease of any group in the country."   —William Castelli, M.D.

"If I could have convinced more slaves that they were slaves,
I could have freed thousands more."   —Harriet Tubman

"Make the most of yourself, for that is all there is of you."
—Ralph Waldo Emerson

RISK FACTOR FOR CANCER

a silver lining

Many people feel that contracting cancer is like losing the lottery. Whatever the causes of cancer—environmental poisons, genetic flaws, or both—many believe that fate plays an enormous role in contracting it. So we are vaguely alarmed that, for some reason, a growing number of us have such bad luck. The idea that toxins in the air, water, food, and general environment might cause cancer has only contributed to our collective sense of powerlessness. After all, we have no choice but to breathe, and we have to eat something. And even though we can pay extra for the privilege of drinking pure distilled water, for most of us this seems like too little, too late.

Although our environment is indeed becoming increasingly toxic, this dark cloud has a silver lining. Most fortunately, in their suspicions regarding the root causes of cancer, it appears that Rachel Carson and other environmentalists may have been only partially correct. After several decades of scientific investigation, the National Cancer Institute has finally been able to determine what types of stressors have the greatest effect on the development of cancer, as shown in the chart below.

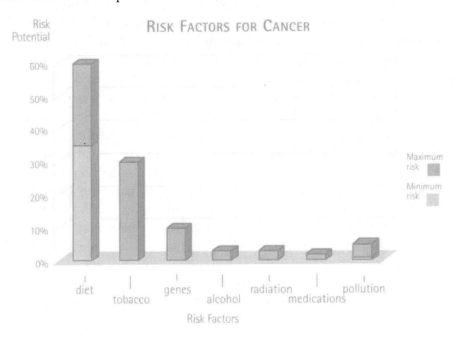

Cancer, it appears, shares an important characteristic with cardio-vascular disease: Its causes can be largely controlled by diet and lifestyle choices. This means that this major threat is largely within our personal control.

The belief that cancer results from exposure to carcinogenic toxins is partially true, but it is extremely misleading. The truth about cancer is more complex, and much more promising. For it appears that the primary culprit in the development of most cancer is observable and controllable: It is the consumption of animal protein. One of the first to grasp this connection was Cornell University biochemist T. Colin Campbell. One of the most respected nutritional biochemists in the world, he discovered that the primary protein of dairy products, casein, appears to be the most aggressive promoter of cancer. For more information on this research go to www.pleasuretrap.com.

Adapted from Lisle, Douglas J., Ph.D., and Goldhamer, Alan, D.C., *The Pleasure Trap*, Healthy Living Publication, Summertown, Tennessee.

At this time, my goal is to help you to feel as good as I do. This is possible only if you become your own doctor. When you begin to listen to your body, you will know what to do and what not to do, what to eat and what not to eat, what to think and what not to think. You will know which emotions are healthy for you, and which are not. For every action there is a reaction. I do not claim to have all the answers, but I have lost the fear that an outside force controls my life. I feel responsible for my own health, for abundance or scarcity, for having loving relationships or unhealthy ones. I know that peace on earth begins with peace within me.

The principles that I share with you in this condensed book, I have learned in my search for wellness. I practice them every day of my life. May they help you to achieve a strong body, a healthy mind, and a loving heart.

—Susana L. Belen

SUMMING UP

1. Detoxify your body.

2. Go organic.

3. Eliminate genetically engineered foods—go to google.com (search engine), key word: GMO (genetically modified organism) or read *GMO Free* by Dr. Mae Wan Ho.

4. Do not use microwaves (see Chapter 9).

5. Buy foods the way they come from nature (fresh, dehydrated, or frozen); avoid packaged foods.

6. Keep portions of staples like rice, beans, lentils, millet, quinoa, noodles, and soups in the freezer, ready to eat.

7. Discover juicing and smoothies.

8. Cook consciously and eat mindfully.

9. Fast one day each week.

10. Control your thoughts (keep them loving and caring).

11. Be good to yourself and your neighbors.

12. Use all your talents in service to mankind.

13. Learn to give.

14. Learn to forgive.

15. Love and respect all of creation—every tree, rock, flower, animal, star, planet, friend, and enemy.

16. Be at peace.

PART II

Food
Preparation
and
Recipes

Cooking is fun!

Make food taste good to you!

9 get organized!

PREPARATION TIPS

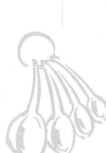

1. Eat at home and shop at health food stores for vegetables and fruits, preferably organically grown.
2. Use purified water for both cooking and drinking.
3. Use stainless steel cookware; NO aluminum cookware, foil, or Teflon-coated cookware; NO microwave cooking.
4. Do your shopping once or twice per week.
5. Soak all fruits and vegetables in a sink full of water and 1 cup of lemon juice or vinegar for 15 minutes; then rinse again with water. Dry them well in spinner and store them in Everfresh bags (they remove damaging gases and prevent the growth of bacteria, fungus, and decay).
6. Have a tray of salad vegetables clean and ready to go.
7. Have another tray ready to go for steamed vegetables.
8. Prepare four dressings of your choice (enough for a week). Use them freely over salads, steamed vegetables, pastas, grains, legumes, baked potatoes, and as dressing for sandwiches.
9. Add oil and BioSalt after the food is cooked (oil and salt should not be heated).
10. Use vegetables and fruits that are fresh or frozen, not canned. Eat raw foods as much as possible. If vegetables are cooked, they should be lightly steamed or baked.
11. Get a Vita-Mix blender. It has long been the most powerful blender one can buy. The Vita-Mix allows you to grind grains, make super smooth smoothies from ice and whole frozen fruit, and even make soups right in the blender because it's so powerful the food heats up as it purees (see pp. 78, 114).
12. Get a Zojirushi Neurofuzzy Rice Cooker. An essential appliance for today's busy schedules, it is the best multipurpose cooker for grains, steamed vegetables, and casseroles. It has a nonstick inner pan that is not Teflon or aluminum. Easy to operate, with a timer you can set so your food is done when you get home; it never burns a meal. (For recipes, see pp. 116–118.)

how to steam your vegetables

It takes practice to be able to steam vegetables so they are tender but not overcooked. In general, steam the harder vegetables, such as potato, sweet potato, beets, yams, and carrots first, then add broccoli and cauliflower, and toward the end add the softer vegetables like mushrooms, zucchini, and leafy greens.

Fill the pan with enough water to be flush with the bottom surface of the steamer (usually to the 1/2-inch or 3/4-inch level). Place the steamer inside and cover until the water boils. Then add the vegetables, cover, and turn the heat to medium. Steam to desired texture.

Emphasize broccoli, zucchini, and string beans in your cleansing diet.

the proven dangers of microwave cooking

Is it possible that millions of people are ignorantly sacrificing their own health in exchange for the convenience of microwave ovens? Why did the Soviet Union ban the use of microwave ovens in 1976? Who invented microwave ovens and why?

The answers to these questions may shock you into throwing your microwave in the trash.

Over 90 percent of American households use microwave ovens for meal preparation. Because microwave ovens are so convenient and energy efficient compared to conventional ovens, very few homes or restaurants are without them. In general, people believe that whatever a microwave oven does, it has no negative effect on either the food cooked in it or on them. Of course, if microwave ovens were really harmful, our government would never allow them on the market, right?

Regardless of what has been *officially* released concerning microwave ovens, we have personally stopped using ours based on the research facts outlined in the report excerpted below. The purpose of this report is to show evidential proof that microwave cooking is neither natural nor healthy, and is far more dangerous to the human body than anyone could imagine. Nevertheless, microwave oven manufacturers and politicians in Washington, aided by plain old inertia on the part of U.S. citizens, have so far successfully suppressed this evidence. As a result, people are continuing to microwave their food in blissful ignorance of the effects and dangers of doing so.

Ten Reasons to Throw Out Your Microwave Oven

The conclusions of the Swiss, Russian, and German scientific clinical studies indicate that we can no longer ignore the microwave ovens sitting in our kitchens.

Based on this research (William P. Kopp, A.R.E.C Research Operations), we will conclude this article with the following:
1. Continually eating food processed from a microwave causes long term, permanent brain damage by "shorting out" electrical impulses in the brain (de-polarizing or de-magnetizing the brain tissue).
2. The human body cannot metabolize (break down) the unknown by-products created in microwave food.
3. Male and female hormone production is shut down and/or altered by continually eating microwaved foods.
4. The effects of microwaved food by-products are residual (long term, permanent) within the human body.

5. Minerals, vitamins, and nutrients of all microwaved food are reduced or altered so that the human body gets little or no benefit, or the human body absorbs altered compounds that cannot be broken down.
6. The minerals in vegetables are altered into cancerous free radicals when cooked in the microwave ovens.
7. Microwaved foods cause stomach and intestinal cancerous growths [tumors]. This may explain the rapidly increased rate of colon cancer in America.
8. The prolonged eating of microwaved foods causes cancerous cells to increase in human blood.
9. Continual ingestion of microwaved food causes immune system deficiencies through lymph gland and blood serum alterations.
10. Eating microwaved food causes loss of memory, concentration, emotional instability, and a decrease in intelligence.

Have you tossed out your microwave oven yet?

For the complete report on the dangers of microwaves, go to www.worldwithoutcancer.com.

forensic research document
Prepared by William P. Kopp
A.R.E.C Research Operations
T061-7R10/10-77F05
Release Priority Class R001a

10 grains, cereals, and legumes

When you are on a vegetarian diet, whole grains and legumes are your staple food. They are a great source of protein, vitamins, and minerals.

good sources of
Protein
Natural Fats
Complex Carbohydrate
B Vitamins
Fiber

WHOLE GRAINS

Quinoa
Millet
Brown rice
Corn
Wheat
Oat
Rye
Buckwheat
Barley
Amaranth
Tritricale
Spelt
Kamut

Whole grains are vegetarians' staple food. They contain B vitamins, minerals, complex carbohydrates, protein, and fiber. Purchase a variety of whole grains and store them in a cool place. Soak them overnight and rinse before cooking.

cooking directions

1 cup grain to $2^1/2$ cups water

Corn meal (polenta) needs 4 cups of water per cup. Cooking time varies from 20 minutes to 1 hour. Bring to a boil, then reduce heat to low and cook until tender. Grains can be served for breakfast or lunch by adding one of the following:

- Nut milk (do not use cow's milk) or nut butter: almond, cashew, or sesame.
- Olive oil and My-Protein.
- Tahini Dressing.
- 4 cups chopped veggies (onions, garlic, parsley, carrots, zucchini, green peas, etc.); cook together and serve.

Save leftover cooked grain to add to salads, soups, or steamed vegetables.

Nut milk

Buy raw organic seeds and nuts (not roasted or salted). Keep them in a cool place.

Soak overnight
2 Tbsp. of each: almonds, pumpkin, sesame, and sunflower seeds

Add
1/2 quart water
vanilla extract, cinnamon, or 1 date to sweeten

Blend and serve over grains. Save leftover nut milk in refrigerator. It is good for three days.

Make a smoothie by using the nut milk and adding a piece of fruit and a few ice cubes.
- To improve flavor, add vanilla extract or carob powder.
- To improve nutrition, add 1 Tbsp. chlorophyll, 1 Tbsp. goat's whey, 1 Tbsp. lecithin, and 1 Tbsp. rice solubles.

Cold mixed cereal
2 cups rolled oats
1/2 cup rolled wheat
1/2 cup rolled rye
1/4 cup chopped raisins
1/4 cup chopped dates
2 Tbsp. honey
1/4 cup oat bran
1/2 cup finely chopped almonds, lightly toasted
1/2 cup finely chopped sesame and sunflower seeds, lightly toasted
1/4 cup finely chopped dried apricots

Stir together all ingredients in a mixing bowl. Transfer to a tightly covered container. Store in a cool place. Serve with nut milk or soy milk. Allow to soak until grains are soft.

Quick hot cereal
1 apple, grated
1/4 cup raisins
1/2 cup grated carrots
(Use leftover pulp from carrot juice.)
1 cup oat bran
2 1/4 cups water

Mix all ingredients in a pan. Bring to a boil, stirring constantly. Lower heat and simmer 3 minutes. Remove from heat. Cover and let stand 5 minutes. Serve with nut milk poured over the cereal.

beans

All beans should be sprouted (soaked in water overnight) before cooking to discourage their tendency to cause gas. When cooking grains and legumes, add chopped vegetables to improve flavor. Cook enough grains and legumes for three or four extra meals; store foods in small containers in your freezer.

LEGUMES

Beans
Garbanzos
Lentils
Peas
Soybeans

NUTS AND SEEDS

Almonds
Sesame seeds
Sunflower seeds
Pumpkin seeds
Cashews
Flax seed
Hemp seed

benefits of hemp

Like other oil seeds, the hemp nut consists mainly of oil (typically 44%), protein (33%), and dietary fiber and other carbohydrates (12%, predominately from residues of the hull). In addition, the nut contains vitamins (particularly the tocopherols and tocotrienols of the vitamin E complex), phytosterols, and trace minerals. Overall, hemp's main nutritional advantage over other seeds lies in the composition of its oil (i.e., its fatty acid profile) and in its protein, which contains all of the essential amino acids in nutritionally significant amounts and in a desirable ratio.

A 1999 workshop by the U.S. National Institute of Health demonstrated the impressive benefits of a balanced omega-6/omega-3 ratio in our diet: reduced risk of arteriosclerosis, sudden cardiac death, and certain types of cancers; decrease in the symptoms of rheumatoid arthritis; mood improvement in bipolar disorders; and optimized development in infants.

11 healthful drinks and smoothies

Let's give our digestive systems a break; let's take a rejuvenation vacation!

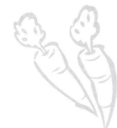

Let's have a fresh vegetable juice every day!

suggested reading:

Dr. N. W. Walker's
Fresh Vegetable and Fruit Juices,
Health Research Books,
Pomeroy, WA, 1981

SUGGESTIONS FOR DAILY EATING

Two solid meals and several liquid meals (every $1^1/_2$ hours) every day. Lots of fresh vegetable juices. Some fresh fruit juices. Herbal teas, lemon water, and smoothies. Following this plan will help your nutrition and elimination. Liquid meals are an instant source of excellent nutrition.

VEGETABLE JUICES

An abundance of fresh, raw juices will help the body release toxins, leaving you energized and healthy. You will begin to see an improvement in your skin and your hair. Many people who have followed the juice therapy have reported increased flexibility in arthritic joints. Colds and flus disappear effortlessly; eyesight improves; and serious illnesses have often improved dramatically.

I recommend the Vita-Mix Total Nutrition Center. It looks like a blender, but it is much more than a blender, operating at 5000 RPM rather than 250 RPM. If you let it run for five minutes, the contents will heat up to the point of boiling. This allows you to make a *hot* raw vegetable soup. It can help you prepare fruit and vegetable juices, vegetable soups, dressings, ice cream, sorbets, smoothies, and nut butters. It also crushes ice, shreds foods instantly, and has an attachment to make bread.

Juice #1
  2 oz. parsley
  6 oz. cucumber
  6 oz. celery
  3 oz. spinach
  6 oz. carrot

Juice #2
  6 oz. carrot
  1 oz. beet
  3 oz. celery

Juice #3
  3 oz. lettuce
  1 oz. beet
  2 oz. celery

Juice #4
  7 oz. celery
  5 oz. lettuce
  4 oz. spinach

Juice #5

6 oz. carrot
2 oz. apple
2 oz. orange
1 oz. lemon

Juice #6

6 oz. grapefruit
3 oz. lemon
7 oz. apple
2 oz. celery

Juice #7

3 oz. carrot
1 oz. beet
1 oz. lemon

Juice #8

1 oz. beet
2 oz. spinach
7 oz. orange

Juice #9

6 oz. grapefruit
3 oz. lemon

Green nut juice

15 almonds soaked overnight in warm water
4 dates pitted and soaked overnight in warm water
5 tsp. sunflower seeds soaked overnight in warm water
16 oz. fresh pineapple juice
2 or 3 handfuls of veggies: spinach, beet tops, dandelion, watercress, endive
1 tsp. bee pollen

Put almonds, dates, sunflower seeds, and 8 oz. fresh pineapple juice in blender and mix. Set aside. Put 8 oz. more fresh pineapple juice in blender, then fill to the top with veggies. Blend all together. Add 1 tsp. bee pollen. Mix the two blends together.

FRUIT DRINKS AND SMOOTHIES

According to Dr. Ann Wigmore, 90 percent of our population has severe digestive problems. In her opinion, blending our food provides an excellent digestive aid. It is a fun way to make delicious after-school smoothies for the kids and for yourself!

Create different smoothies by changing the fruit or the fruit juice, or by adding soy milk or rice milk.
1. Apple juice, banana, strawberries, ice
2. Apple juice, cantaloupe, watermelon, banana, ice
3. Banana, nut milk, soy milk or kefir, strawberries, ice (sweeten with stevia)
4. Banana, mango, orange juice, ice
5. Tropical fruit juice, raspberries, boysenberries, peaches

For a more nutritional drink, add one or several of the following ingredients:
- 1 Tbsp. chlorophyll
- 1 Tbsp. lecithin
- 1 Tbsp. goat's whey
- 1 Tbsp. rice bran solubles
- 1 Tbsp. fiber

To improve flavor add 1/4 tsp. vanilla and/or 1 Tbsp. carob powder.

Café Latte

To a cup of hot water, add:
1 Tbsp. goat's whey
1 Tbsp. probiotics powder
Dash of carob powder
1/4 tsp. vanilla

Mix and drink as a coffee replacement. For a more decorative look, pour this mixture into a blender for a few seconds, then serve.

12 dressings

Dressings are fun to prepare and add flavor to your food. Once a week, prepare three or four different dressings, enough to last for the whole week. The same dressing can be used over salads, steamed vegetables, brown rice, noodles, and sandwiches.

Lemon garlic dressing

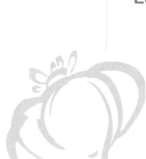

juice of a lemon
1 clove garlic
1 clove
1 yellow onion
1 tsp. oregano
1/2 tsp. kelp
olive oil (optional)

Mix in blender. Allow flavors to blend in refrigerator.

Italian herbal dressing

3 large tomatoes
1/2 peeled cucumber
1 yellow onion
1 clove garlic
dash of cayenne
1 tsp. dill
2 Tbsp. lemon juice
olive oil (optional)

Mix above ingredients in a blender. Chill to allow flavors to blend.

Avocado green dressing

2 tsp. salty liquid seasoning, season to taste
1 medium avocado, ripened
juice of 1/2 lemon
1 clove garlic
1 pinch cayenne (optional)

Mix in blender.

"Kelp from the sea" dressing

2–3 Tbsp. lemon juice
1 clove garlic

1 yellow onion
1/2 tsp. kelp
1/2 tsp. salty liquid seasoning
1 tsp. oregano

Mix in blender. Allow flavors to blend in refrigerator.

Dynamic herbal dressing

2/3 cup lemon juice
3 scallions
1/4 cup parsley
1/3 tsp. each oregano and rosemary
1/2 tsp. cayenne
1/2 tsp. celery seed
1/2 tsp. basil

Mix in blender and chill for 1 hour before serving.

Cleansing chili sauce

3 tomatoes
1 green pepper
1/2 tsp. oregano
1/8 tsp. cayenne
1/4 cup green onions
1–2 tsp. chili powder

Put all ingredients in blender or food processor. Blend until tomatoes and pepper are chopped coarse.

Tahini dressing

12 oz. tahini sesame butter (raw)
juice from 3 lemons
1/2 cup salty liquid seasoning
dash of garlic, cayenne, kelp

Mix well in blender. Keep refrigerated. Delicious over brown rice, noodles, salads, and soups, or as spread for sandwiches and steamed vegetables.

Special sauce for steamed vegetables

a handful of sunflower seed sprouts
a handful of buckwheat sprouts
1/2 avocado
1/2 cup lemon juice
4 Tbsp. sesame tahini
4 Tbsp. salty liquid seasoning
garlic, vegetable seasoning, cayenne

Blend and pour over steamed vegetables.

Healthful green dressing

juice from 2 lemons
1 cup water
1 red onion
fresh green chilies, seeds removed
1 small bunch cilantro
1 pinch cayenne
2 cloves garlic
1 small bunch parsley

Blend until chopped coarse. Use as salad dressing or turn into Wholly Guacamole.

Wholly guacamole

2 medium avocados, ripe
Healthful Green Dressing

Smash avocado with fork, mix in Healthful Green Dressing. Serve on top of vegetable salad, use in place of salad dressing or as a dip for celery stalks, or serve over noodles or rice.

Healthful mayonnaise

1 cup raw cashews
juice of 1 lemon
garlic, cayenne

Soak cashews overnight in 1/3 cup water. Grind cashews in blender and add lemon juice, garlic, and cayenne. Store in a jar and serve as mayonnaise.

Chinese ginger sauce

2 cloves garlic
2 green onions, chopped
2 cups water
2 Tbsp. arrowroot dissolved in 4 Tbsp. water
1 tsp. oil
1 Tbsp. ginger, minced
1 Tbsp. olive oil
4 Tbsp. salty liquid seasoning

Sauté garlic, ginger, and onion in a little water. Add remaining water. Bring to a boil. Add liquid seasoning. Stir in arrowroot to thicken mixture and add oil. Serve over steamed vegetables, tofu, or rice.

13 salads

Salads contain lots of enzymes, vitamins, and minerals. They are very nutritional, easy to prepare, and fun to decorate.

VEGETABLES

Eat a large variety of the following vegetables daily: alfalfa and other sprouts, artichokes, arugula, asparagus, beets, broccoli, brussels sprouts, cabbage (red or green), carrots, cauliflower, celery, chard, corn, cucumbers, dill, eggplants, garlic, kale, kohlrabi, lettuce (bibb, leaf, romaine—not iceberg), okra, onions, parsley, parsnips, peas, peppers, radishes, scallions, spinach, string beans, squash, tomatoes, and zucchini.

Summer green salad

In a jar, shake well:

4 Tbsp. oil
1/3 cup lemon juice
dash BioSalt or sea salt
1/4 cup basil, finely chopped
1/8 cup fresh dill, finely chopped

In a large salad bowl, layer:

4 cups lettuce, spinach, and/or chard, torn into small pieces
1 cup mustard greens, torn into small pieces
1 large tomato, cut into wedges
4 scallions, diced
1½ cups mushrooms, sliced thin
1 avocado, diced
1/2 cup almonds, soaked 24 hours and cut in half

Pour dressing over salad and toss. Serves 4

Avocado salad

In a medium-sized salad bowl, layer:

1 avocado, cut into cubes
2 tomatoes, cut into chunks
1 bell pepper, cut in short slivers
1 cup mushrooms, sliced
1/2 cup sunflower seeds, soaked 12 hours

Pour dressing over salad and toss. Serves 2

Gourmet cold salad

Grind in blender or food processor:

1 package frozen peas
2 green onions
2 fresh small carrots
1/4 cup tahini dressing or Healthful Green Dressing

Mix to make into a thick paste. Serve a scoop on a lettuce leaf and pour dressing over it, or fill a whole wheat pita pocket as a sandwich. Serves 6

salad suggestions

It is a good idea to keep marinated veggies in the refrigerator to spruce up an ordinary salad. Vegetables should be very lightly steamed before putting them in a vinaigrette (preferred substitute is lemon or lime juice). A good rule of thumb is five minutes, but this does vary. Suggested vinaigrette vegetables: string beans, cauliflower, broccoli, asparagus.

Vinaigrette

1 cup of unpasteurized apple cider vinegar
1/3 cup olive oil

Here is a quick list of some simple but very tasty salads.

1. Beets with Cloves
   Steam beets. Drain. Slice in chunks. Marinate with ground cloves, oil, vinegar, and lime juice.
2. Sprouts
   Raw sprouts with lime juice, pepper, dried tomatoes, onions, and a dash of liquid seasoning.
3. Grated Carrots
   Raw, grated carrots marinated in orange and lime juices and sprinkled with cinnamon.
4. Celery
   Celery and lime juice with a dash of Healthful Mayonnaise.
5. Diced Pineapple and Shredded Cabbage
   Diced pineapple, shredded cabbage, lime juice, and raisins.
6. Watercress and Mushrooms
   Watercress and mushrooms in vinaigrette.
7. Sliced Cucumber
   Sliced cucumbers with dill weed and lime juice.

8. **Steamed Carrots**
   Steamed carrots with dill weed, lemon, or lime juice.
9. **Jicama**
   Jicama slices, sprinkled with lime juice and paprika.
10. **Rice and Lentil Salad**
    Toss leftover cooked rice or leftover cooked lentils with chopped raw onions, chopped tomatoes, and enough vinaigrette to flavor.

Fresh corn salad

2 ears of fresh corn
2 tomatoes, chopped
1/2 onion, chopped
1/4 cup chopped parsley
2–3 jalapeno chilies, chopped
2 Tbsp. vinegar
4 Tbsp. olive oil

Slice corn kernels off of the cob. Boil until tender. (If corn is very fresh, use it raw.) Drain well. Toss with chopped tomatoes, onions, parsley, several finely chopped jalapeno chilies, and the vinegar marinade. Also excellent with cold beans tossed in it. Serves 2

Cucumber salad

6 cucumbers
8 oz. kefir
2 cloves garlic, crushed
1 Tbsp. dill weed
2 Tbsp. lemon or lime juice
1/4 tsp. tumeric (optional)

Peel cucumbers and score. Slice thinly in rounds and marinate in mixture of kefir, garlic, dill weed, and lime juice. You may add tumeric for an interesting flavor, but it will color the mixture yellow. Serves 4

Potato salad

6 baked or broiled potatoes, diced
2 grated carrots
1 cup diced celery
2 Tbsp. finely diced onions
2 tsp. celery seed
1 package fresh or frozen peas, cooked

1/3 cup chopped parsley
3 Tbsp. lime juice
1 tsp. mustard powder
1 tsp. rosemary
6 Tbsp. Healthful Mayonnaise
6 Tbsp. Healthful Green Dressing

Mix all ingredients and chill well before serving. Serves 4

Spaghetti squash salad

1 spaghetti squash (about 2^1/$_2$ lb.)
8 cherry tomatoes, quartered
1 green bell pepper, chopped
4 scallions, sliced
1 cup Wholly Guacamole dressing

Preheat oven to 350 degrees. Prick squash with fork and bake for 45 minutes to 1 hour, until shell is easily depressed when touched with spoon. Cut squash in half, and remove seeds and stringy flesh. With a fork, gently scrape remaining flesh to remove spaghetti-like strands of squash. In a large salad bowl, combine squash, tomatoes, green peppers, and scallions. Toss with Wholly Guacamole and season to taste. Serves 2

Zucchini salad

3 zucchinis
1 tomato, chopped
1 onion, sliced
1 clove garlic, minced
3 Tbsp. olive oil
dash BioSalt and cayenne
lettuce leaves
2 carrots, shredded
6 radishes, sliced
1 cucumber, sliced
4 Tbsp. olives
2 Tbsp. parsley, chopped

Lightly steam zucchini. Let it cool, then chop zucchini and place in a large mixing bowl. Add tomatoes, onions, garlic, and mix gently. Add olive oil, BioSalt, and cayenne. Mix and refrigerate for two hours. To serve, line a serving platter with lettuce leaves and scoop the zucchini mixture on top. Arrange carrots, radishes, cucumbers, and olives around the edges. Garnish with parsley. Serves 4

Ginger salad

2 cups broccoli, chopped
3 cups carrots, shredded
1 cooked sweet potato, cooled and cubed
1 red pepper, sliced
4 Tbsp. lemon juice
2 tsp. ginger powder
1/2 cup Healthful Mayonnaise
1 cup raisins

Combine broccoli and carrots. Add sweet potato and pepper. Place in large bowl and toss with lemon juice. Toss again with ginger powder, mayonnaise, and raisins before serving. Serves 4

Antipasto salad

1 lb. firm tofu, diced
1 cup celery sliced
1/2 cup mushrooms, sliced
1/2 red pepper, sliced
2 medium tomatoes, chopped
6 Tbsp. Wholly Guacamole dressing

Mix the tofu and vegetables in a large bowl. Pour dressing over them and mix gently. Marinate in the refrigerator for 1 hour before serving. Serves 4

Tomato salad

1 onion, sliced
1/4 cup apple cider vinegar
6 Tbsp. olive oil
Healthful Green Dressing
6 medium tomatoes, thickly sliced
6 oz. goat cheese (grated)

Place sliced onion in a mixing bowl. In a saucepan, bring the vinegar just to a boil. Pour it over the onion. Let sit until cool, then drain the vinegar. Blend olive oil and Healthful Green Dressing together. Place tomato slices on each serving plate. Arrange onion slices on top of tomatoes and sprinkle with cheese. Serve 1 Tbsp. Healthful Green Dressing and olive oil mixture over each tomato. Serves 4

Salad florentine

3 cups Boston lettuce
3 cups spinach
4 potatoes, cooked, cooled, and cubed
2 cups green beans, cooked
1 cup carrots, cooked, cooled, and cubed
1 sliced and peeled cucumber
1 cup red bell pepper strips
1/2 cup olives
1 cup cherry tomatoes, halved
Wholly Guacamole dressing

On a large serving plate, arrange lettuce and spinach leaves. Top with rows of potatoes, green beans, carrots, cucumbers, and bell peppers. Add olives and tomatoes. Serve with Wholly Guacamole dressing. Serves 4

Beans-vegetable salad

6 cups escarole
2 cups romaine
2 cups white beans, cooked
2 cups red beans, cooked
1¹/₂ cups diced celery
1¹/₂ cups cherry tomato, halved
1 cup sliced zucchini
1/2 sliced onion
1/2 cup fresh cilantro, chopped
1/2 cup fresh parsley, chopped
"Kelp from the Sea" Dressing

In a big salad bowl, mix all ingredients. Add "Kelp from the Sea" Dressing. Serves 4

Cooked beet salad

6 beets
1/4 cabbage
1 carrot
Tahini Dressing

Steam beets, then cool. Scoop out centers. Shred cabbage and carrot, and mix with chopped beet centers. Mix with Tahini Dressing. Fill beet cups with mixture and chill. Serve on spinach leaves. Serves 4

Rice salad

1 yam, cubed
1 cup cauliflower
1 cup broccoli
2 cups brown rice, cooked
1 cup firm tofu, mashed
5 Tbsp. salty liquid seasoning
1 cup water
1/2 cup fresh parsley, chopped
4 Tbsp. Tahini Dressing

Steam yam, cauliflower, and broccoli until tender. Set aside. Mix rice with vegetables. Blend tofu with Tahini Dressing, liquid seasoning, water, and parsley in small saucepan. Heat for 5 minutes. Let it cool, then pour over rice and vegetables. Chill and serve. Serves 4

Winter salad

1/2 lb. tofu, cut into cubes
4 Tbsp. olive oil
1 Tbsp. dill seed
1/4 cup lemon juice
dash BioSalt or sea salt
$2^{1}/2$ cups cabbage, finely shredded
$1^{1}/2$ cups carrots, grated
3/4 cup radish, red and/or daikon, sliced thin
1/2 cup onions, diced
1 tomato, cut
1/2 cup sunflower seeds, soaked 12 hours

Whip marinade ingredients together in a bowl with wire whisk: olive oil, dill seed, lemon juice, and salt. Pour over tofu and marinate for 1 hour or more, stirring occasionally. In a large salad bowl, toss cabbage, carrots, radish, onions, tomato, and sunflower seeds. Pour tofu and marinade over salad and toss. Serves 4

Spinach tofu salad

1/2 lb. tofu, cut into cubes
4 Tbsp. olive oil
2 Tbsp. salty liquid seasoning
4 Tbsp. lemon juice
1 tsp. curry powder
5 cups spinach, torn into small pieces
$1^{1}/_{2}$ cups mushrooms, sliced thin and halved
1 cup mung bean sprouts
3/4 cup red radish and/or daikon, sliced
4 scallions, diced

To make marinade, shake well in a jar: olive oil, liquid seasoning, lemon juice, and curry powder. Pour over tofu and marinate for 1 hour or more, stirring occasionally.

In a large bowl, toss spinach, mushrooms, mung bean sprouts, radish, and scallions. Pour marinated tofu over salad and toss.
Serves 4

14 soups

Nothing like soup on a cold day! So easy to prepare. Cook some extra and save it in your freezer.

Cleansing mixed-green soup

1 medium turnip, diced
1 small rutabaga, diced
1 carrot, scraped and diced
1 medium beet, diced
3 quarts water
1 small bunch greens of your choice
1/4 head red cabbage, shredded
1 small bunch turnip greens
1/4 tsp. fresh cracked pepper
1 small zucchini, diced
1 stalk celery, chopped
1/4 tsp. marjoram
1/4 tsp. oregano
dash cayenne
1 onion, diced
1/2 lb. fresh broccoli
1 bay leaf
1/4 tsp. basil
salty liquid seasoning

Place turnip, rutabaga, carrot, and beet in a deep soup pot with water. Simmer, covered, until the vegetables are partially tender. Then add all of the remaining ingredients and simmer, covered, for approximately 4 minutes. Place steamed vegetables and water in a blender, add liquid seasoning to taste, and serve. Serves 8 to 10

Susana's super soup

1/2 potato
1/2 carrot
1/2 onion
1/2 sweet potato
3 quarts water
1/2 cup beet leaves
1 zucchini
1 cup celery
dash salty liquid seasoning
dash olive oil
1–2 cloves garlic, chopped
dash kelp
dash cayenne

Steam potato, carrot, onion, and sweet potato. When almost done, add beet leaves, zucchini, celery. Blend steamed vegetables and water until slightly puréed. Add liquid seasoning, olive oil, garlic, kelp, and cayenne to season. Serves 6

Winter hearty soup

1/2 cup white lima beans
1/2 cup split peas
1 sweet potato, diced
1 large onion, chopped
1 bunch cilantro, chopped
1 bunch parsley, chopped
1 cup carrot pulp
dash salty liquid seasoning
pinch garlic, kelp, cayenne

Soak lima beans and split peas overnight and drain. Add fresh water and then add sweet potato, onion, cilantro, parsley, and carrot pulp. Cook slowly. Add seasoning to taste. Serves 8

Quick energy soup

In blender, place the following ingredients (all raw):
1¹/₂ cups water
1 medium organic carrot, chopped
1 organic apple, cored and chopped
1/2 medium onion
1 small handful of dulse (purplish seaweed)

Blend for about 15 seconds, and then add:
1 medium zucchini, chopped
1/2 stalk of celery
1/4 tsp. basil leaves
3 Tbsp. salty liquid seasoning
dash cayenne

Blend for 15 seconds, and then add:
1 medium avocado
1 small handful freshly cut lettuce or greens
(try something out of the ordinary—
like buckwheat greens)
1 small handful freshly cut sunflower sprouts

Blend for 15 seconds and serve. Serves 4

Asparagus soup

1 medium onion, diced
2 celery stalks, diced
1 lb. asparagus, chopped
1 medium potato, diced
dash cayenne pepper
dash BioSalt
1/4 tsp. tarragon
1/2 tsp. parsley
1/4 tsp. rosemary
2 quarts water
2 Tbsp. olive oil
1/4 cup chopped cilantro

In a large soup pot, sauté the onions and celery until tender, about 3 to 5 minutes. Add asparagus, potato, cayenne, BioSalt, and herbs. Add enough water to cover the vegetables. Bring to a boil, lower heat, and simmer for 25 to 30 minutes until the vegetables are tender. Remove from heat, and cool for 5 minutes. Purée the vegetables in small batches in a blender, returning each batch to the soup pot. Serve immediately with a garnish of chopped cilantro. Add oil and BioSalt at serving time. Serves 4

Bean soup

1 onion, chopped
1 carrot, chopped
1 stalk celery, chopped
2 cups cooked beans (choose from black, navy or great white northern, red, pinto, fava, kidney, lima, moong, adzuki beans, or a mixture)
8 cups water
fresh basil
1/2 tsp. oregano
pinch cayenne
pinch garlic powder
1 Tbsp. olive oil
dash salty liquid seasoning

Sauté onion, carrot, and celery in a little water. Add 1 cup of beans and water. Purée the remaining beans and 1 cup of water in a blender. Stir in the remaining ingredients. Bring to a boil, lower heat, and simmer for 15 minutes. Serve and add olive oil and liquid seasoning. Serves 4

Each variety of bean has unique nutritional properties. Black beans and small red beans are not only high in protein, carbohydrates, folate, calcium, and fiber, they have more antioxidant activity, gram for gram, than other beans, followed by brown, yellow, and white beans. They are a rich but overlooked source of antioxidants and may provide health benefits similar to grapes and cranberries. Although only dry beans were used in the study, frozen or canned beans are thought to have similar antioxidant activity.

From the June 9 print edition of the *Journal of Agricultural and Food Chemistry*, a peer-reviewed publication of the American Chemical Society, the world's largest scientific society.

15 main dishes

TOFU: "MEAT WITHOUT THE BONE"

Low in calories, high in good-quality protein, and rich in both calcium and iron, tofu is ideal for weight watchers. An 8-ounce serving contains 147 to 164 calories. You may want to limit your intake of tofu because of its potentially unhealthy effect on estrogen levels.

Tofu spread

12 oz. tofu
1$\frac{1}{2}$ bananas
2 Tbsp. lemon juice
2 Tbsp. honey
1/3 cup almond butter (optional)

Combine all ingredients in a blender and purée until smooth. Serve on seven-grain bread and top with nuts, raisins, or sliced bananas. Serves 10

Tofu-avocado spread

8 oz. tofu
1 avocado
2 Tbsp. Healthful Mayonnaise
1 pinch cayenne, garlic, and kelp
2 Tbsp. salty liquid seasoning

Mix all ingredients in blender. Serve with raw vegetables. Serves 5

Tofu, carrot, raisin, and walnut salad

6 oz. tofu, well drained
1 cup grated carrots
1/2 cup raisins
1/2 cup walnuts, diced
1$\frac{1}{2}$ Tbsp. miso
2 tsp. honey
1 tsp. lemon juice
2 Tbsp. sesame butter
4 lettuce leaves

Wrap tofu in a cloth towel, squeeze out the water, and let it sit for 15 minutes until firm. Mash well. Combine with rest of the ingredients and mix well. Serve on lettuce or in sandwiches. Serves 2

Tofu-pita pizza

Use tofu, soy cheese, fresh tomatoes, cayenne, garlic, kelp, fresh oregano, and basil.

Stuff pita with all ingredients and bake in the oven for 15 minutes.

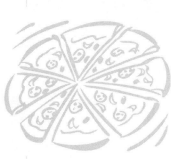

Tofu and onions

2 onions
8 oz. tofu
pinch garlic powder, cayenne, kelp
2 Tbsp. salty liquid seasoning
2 Tbsp. olive oil

Chop onions and sauté in water. Chop tofu into cubes and add to onions. Add garlic, cayenne, kelp; cover and simmer. Allow to cook for a few minutes, then remove from heat. Add liquid seasoning and olive oil, and serve over steamed vegetables. Serves 2

PASTA

Pasta is low in calories and fat, and rich in complex carbohydrates. It is easy to make and is used in an endless variety of recipes. Read labels for whole-grain pastas. No white, enriched, bleached, or unbleached flour.

Boil pasta according to instructions and drain. Add one of the following seasonings:

1. Olive oil and salty liquid seasoning like Quick Sip, Bragg's Liquid Aminos, We Care My-Protein. Season with cayenne, garlic, kelp, and chopped cilantro.
2. Tahini Dressing
3. Healthful Tomato Sauce
4. Wholly Guacamole

Pasta deliciosa

2 Tbsp. Wholly Guacamole
2 Tbsp. Tahini Dressing
1 Tbsp. olive oil
3 Tbsp. salty liquid seasoning
1 pinch cayenne, garlic, and kelp
2 Tbsp. nut milk

Stir ingredients together and serve over 8 ounces of hot cooked pasta.

Pasta
Look for artichoke, brown rice, oat, corn, spelt, whole durham flour, quinoa, etc.

Healthful tomato sauce

4 large red onions, chopped
6 carrots, grated
4 fresh tomatoes, chopped
3 zucchini, chopped
1 red bell pepper, chopped
3 cloves of garlic
1/2 cup parsley, chopped
1/2 cup cilantro, chopped

In a pan, boil 1/2 cup water and sauté the above ingredients. Cover and simmer for an hour. At serving time, add the following ingredients and pour over 12 oz. package of cooked penne. Serves 6

2 Tbsp. olive oil
2 Tbsp. salty liquid seasoning
pinch cayenne, garlic, and kelp

Pasta al olio (garlic-oil-parsley)

1 package (8 oz.) pasta
6 Tbsp. olive oil
3 cloves garlic
whole cayenne peppers
1 bunch parsley, as finely cut as possible
Vegan parmesan cheese, freshly grated

Cook pasta and drain. While pasta is cooking, sauté garlic pieces and cayenne peppers in olive oil until golden brown. Add sautéed garlic, cayenne peppers, and parsley to drained pasta and toss. Sprinkle with Vegan parmesan cheese. Serves 4

Papaya noodles

1 package (1 lb.) medium-sized pasta such as penne or shells
6 Tbsp. olive oil
dash cayenne
1 papaya, peeled, seeded, and chopped
1 cup cherry tomatoes, halved
1 bunch green onions, thinly sliced
1 yellow bell pepper, seeded and chopped
1 cucumber, quartered lengthwise and sliced
6 Tbsp. rice vinegar
1 small jalapeno pepper, finely minced
2 Tbsp. chopped fresh cilantro or parsley

Cook pasta. Drain and transfer to medium-sized bowl; add oil and season with cayenne to taste. Cool to room temperature. Add papaya, tomatoes, sliced green onions, bell pepper, and cucumber, and toss together. In small bowl, combine vinegar, jalapeno pepper, and cilantro. Add to pasta and toss to combine. Refrigerate 1 to 2 hours or until chilled. To serve, garnish with green onion brushes. Serves 8

Basil-pesto pasta

3 cloves garlic
2 cups fresh basil
1/4 cup pine nuts
1/4 cup olive oil
1/3 cup goat cheese
1 (8 oz.) box pasta

Blend garlic, basil, pine nuts, and olive oil for 2 to 3 minutes. Add cheese and blend for 1 more minute. Boil pasta and drain. Add pesto mixture and serve. Make extra pesto sauce and refrigerate. Serves 4

Bow ties with greens and mushrooms

1 package (8 oz.) bow tie noodles
3 Tbsp. olive oil
3 green onions, chopped
3/4 cup sliced mushrooms
1 rib celery, thinly sliced
dash finely grated, peeled ginger root
1 lb. kale, spinach, or other dark leafy green, rinsed and broken into small pieces (tough stalks removed)
dash BioSalt or sea salt
3/4 cup water
2 Tbsp. arrowroot powder
1/4 cup cold water
1/4 cup grated goat cheese

Cook pasta and drain. Meanwhile, in large skillet over medium heat, heat oil. Add green onions, mushrooms, celery, and ginger. Cook 2 to 3 minutes, stirring constantly; do not brown. Add kale and 3/4 cup water. Cover; reduce heat to low, and cook about 15 minutes or until vegetables are tender-crisp. In small bowl, mix arrowroot powder with cold water; stir into vegetable mixture and cook just until heated through. To serve, toss vegetables with hot pasta in medium-sized bowl and sprinkle with shredded goat cheese and BioSalt. Serves 4

Use your imagination to mix an endless variety of vegetables, grains, seeds, and nuts.

Anchovy pasta

1 package (1 lb.) spaghetti
1 Tbsp. olive oil
3 garlic cloves, thinly sliced
1/4 Tbsp. red pepper flakes
6 anchovy fillets, finely chopped
1 jar (6^1/$_2$ oz.) oil-cured olives, pitted
3 large, ripe tomatoes, chopped
dash cayenne
fresh cilantro (optional)

Cook pasta; drain. Meanwhile, in large skillet over medium heat, heat oil. Stir in garlic, pepper flakes, and anchovies; cook 1 minute. Add olives and tomatoes; cook 8 to 10 minutes or until sauce thickens, stirring occasionally. Season with cayenne to taste. To serve, toss pasta with sauce in large bowl, garnish with cilantro, and serve immediately. Serves 4

Radish leaf delight pasta

1 package (8 oz.) linguini or other long, thin pasta
3 bunches radish leaves, washed well
6 Tbsp. olive oil
dash cayenne pepper
dash BioSalt or sea salt
4 Tbsp. goat cheese, freshly grated

Cook pasta and radish leaves together; drain. Place back into the pan, add olive oil and cayenne pepper; toss to combine. Sprinkle with cheese. Serves 4

Linguini with broccoli and feta

1 package (8 oz.) linguini or other long, thin pasta
2 bunches broccoli, cut into small florets (stems removed)
2 Tbsp. oil
2 large garlic cloves, minced
5 green onions, thinly sliced
1^1/$_2$ Tbsp. chopped fresh thyme or 1/2 tsp. dried thyme leaves
4 oz. feta cheese or soft goat cheese
dash cayenne
dash BioSalt or sea salt

Cook pasta and drain. Meanwhile, steam broccoli florets about 3 minutes or just until tender-crisp; set aside. In large skillet over medium-high heat, heat oil. Add garlic and green onions; cook about 1 minute or until tender but not brown, stirring often. Add thyme and reserved broccoli; cook 2 minutes longer, stirring often. Remove from heat; add feta cheese. Transfer mixture to large bowl; add hot pasta and toss together. To serve, season with cayenne to taste. Serves 4

Summer dream pasta

1 package (8 oz.) spaghetti or other pasta
5–7 garlic cloves, finely cut
4 tomatoes, cut into finger-tip-sized pieces
1 bunch parsley, finely cut
juice of 1 lemon
dash cayenne pepper
dash BioSalt or sea salt
8 Tbsp. goat cheese, freshly grated

Cook pasta and drain. While pasta is cooking, place lemon juice, cayenne pepper, BioSalt, garlic cloves, tomatoes, and parsley into a bowl and stir until well mixed. Add this mixture to drained pasta. Sprinkle with parmesan cheese. Serve hot or cold. Serves 4

Lasagna

1 package lasagna noodles
1 package tofu
1 package soy cheese
1 package goat cheese
Healthful Tomato Sauce

Boil noodles and drain carefully. In a rectangular pan, alternate: one layer Healthful Tomato Sauce, one layer lasagna noodles, one layer grated cheese and tofu. Continue layers until pan is almost full. Bake at 350 degrees for 30 minutes. Serve with green salad. Serves 8

OTHER DISHES

Vegetable loaf
carrots
broccoli
summer squash
jicama
cauliflower
cucumber
yellow squash
onion
cashew butter
tahini butter
vegetable seasoning (optional)

Grate all the raw vegetables above or add your own favorites (use amount of vegetables appropriate to your family size). In a bowl, combine enough cashew butter with a little tahini to make mixture stick together. You may want to add a bit of vegetable seasoning. Mix with grated vegetables. Press mixture into small individual loaf pans; turn out onto a plate lined with sprouts and sliced tomatoes.

Sunburgers
2 medium carrots, grated
1 onion, chopped fine
1 tsp. parsley
1/2 cup oatmeal
1/8 tsp. sweet basil
1 cup celery, chopped fine
1 fresh tomato, chopped
dash BioSalt or sea salt
1 cup sunflower seeds, ground

Mix all ingredients raw. Form into patties. Bake 30 minutes at 350 degrees. May need turning halfway through baking time.
Serves 2

Creamy eggplant casserole

1 large eggplant
3 cups brown rice, cooked
1 green pepper
1 medium onion
2 cups raw cashews
1 cup water
dash BioSalt or sea salt
1/2 tsp. celery salt
1/4 tsp. garlic salt
1/2 tsp. sage
3 Tbsp. parsley
2–4 almonds, cut

Cube eggplant. Boil until tender (do not overcook). Chop pepper and onion and sauté over low heat in water. Whiz 1 cup water with cashews in blender; blend until smooth. Drain eggplant and add onion and pepper. Stir until eggplant is slightly mashed. Add rice, cashew mixture, and seasoning. Blend well. Pour into casserole, sprinkle with almonds, and bake for 1 hour at 325 degrees. Serves 4

Millet tomato loaf

1 cup tomato juice
1 cup millet, uncooked
1/2 cup olives, chopped
1 medium onion, quartered
dash BioSalt or sea salt
1/2 tsp. sage
1/2 tsp. savory
5 cups fresh tomatoes
1/2 cup nuts or seeds

In a 2-quart casserole dish, combine tomato juice with millet and olives, and soak overnight. Blend smooth the remaining ingredients. Stir all ingredients into casserole. Cover and bake at 350 degrees for 1 hour and 20 minutes. Remove from oven, take lid off, and let set 10 minutes before serving. Serves 6

Split pea stew

1¹/₂ cups dry split peas
6 cups water
2 tomatoes, chopped
1 red pepper, chopped
1 onion, chopped
2 cloves garlic, chopped
1/4 cup chopped parsley and cilantro
2 cups cubed sweet potatoes
2 cups carrot pulp
2 cups small broccoli florets
chopped parsley for garnish
4 Tbsp. salty liquid seasoning

Soak split peas overnight. Bring split peas and soaking water to a boil. Add tomatoes. Simmer, covered, until peas are very soft (30 minutes). In a blender or food processor, purée pea mixture until smooth, adding a little extra water if necessary. Return puréed peas to a saucepan. Cover and keep warm.

In a large, deep pot, combine onion, garlic, parsley, cilantro, sweet potatoes, and the remaining 2 cups water. Bring to a boil, reduce heat, and simmer 6 to 7 minutes. Add broccoli and carrots, and simmer another 6 to 8 minutes or until broccoli is tender. Add pea mixture, reduce heat to low, cover, and cook gently. Serve and garnish with parsley, cilantro, and liquid seasoning. Serves 8

Zucchini casserole with grains

1 cup rice (or other grain), cooked
2 zucchinis, sliced thinly
1 eggplant, sliced thinly
2 carrots, sliced in circles
1 onion, sliced in circles
6 cloves garlic, crushed
1 tomato, sliced in 1/2-inch circles
1 cup raw sliced celery
3/4 cup raw almonds,
sesame seeds, sunflower seeds
oregano, basil, and parsley
1 cup grated or cubed soy cheese

When zucchini, eggplant, carrots, celery, and onion are sliced, steam each separately (or keep separate in a steamer) for approximately 5 minutes. Remove from heat. Lightly oil large casserole dish. Put a thin layer of grain mixture on the bottom of the dish, and add successive layers of zucchini, eggplant, onions, almonds and seeds, oregano, carrots, celery, basil, parsley, and so on, until top of casserole is reached. Top with sliced tomatoes and sprinkle with grated cheese substitute like Tofurella and sesame seeds. Bake covered for 45 minutes at 450 degrees. Serves 4

Sweet potato sticks

2 large sweet potatoes
1/2 cup sesame seeds
1 Tbsp. sesame oil

Boil sweet potatoes until soft but not mushy. Let cool or refrigerate overnight. Peel and cut potatoes into pieces about $2^{1}/_{2}$" x 1/2". Roll potato sticks in sesame seeds, pressing to make seeds stick. Sauté in oil for 1 minute on each side, drain, and cool. Serve cool or broil briefly and serve hot. Serves 2

Chop suey

2 zucchini
2 yellow squash
2 onions, chopped
3 celery stalks, sliced
3 cups Chinese peapods
1 cup sprouts (bean or lentil)
6 Tbsp. olive oil
5 Tbsp. salty liquid seasoning
3 green onions, chopped
ground almonds

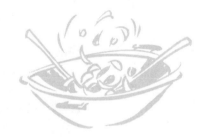

Put 1/2 cup water in pan and heat. Add sliced zucchini, yellow squash, onions, celery, and Chinese peas. Sauté briefly at low heat. Do not overcook. Just before removing from heat, add sprouts. Turn off heat and let stand about 5 minutes. Add olive oil and liquid seasoning. Serve over rice, garnish with green onions, and sprinkle with ground almonds. Serves 4

Baked sweet potatoes

12 sweet potatoes
1/2 cup nut milk
3 apples, chopped
1/2 cup almonds, chopped

Boil sweet potatoes and let chill. Remove top lengthwise from each potato, cutting off no more then one quarter of the potato. Scoop out insides of potatoes without breaking the skin. Place the contents in a blender, adding nut milk, apples, and almonds until the consistency is creamy. Spoon mixture back into potato skins. Heat on top rack of oven at 250 degrees for 45 minutes. Serves 12

Sweet and sour cabbage

1 carrot
1 small cabbage
2 apples
1 pint water
1/3 cup lemon juice
2 Tbsp. date crystals
dash BioSalt or sea salt
3 cloves
3 Tbsp. olive oil

Shred cabbage and carrot. Put 1/2 cup water in saucepan and add shredded vegetables. Shred apples, and mix with water, lemon juice, date crystals, and cloves. Pour over grated vegetables and cook at low temperature until tender. Add olive oil and BioSalt before serving. Serves 4

Vegetable noodle casserole

1 package of De Boles noodles (8 oz.)
4 cups chopped vegetables: celery, onions, red peppers,
water chestnuts, parsley
3 Tbsp. olive oil
1¹/₂ cups water
3 Tbsp. Tahini Dressing

Boil noodles until tender. Strain. Sauté vegetables (in a little water) until tender. Add noodles, and stir lightly with a fork. Add remaining water, oil, and Tahini Dressing and serve.

Eggplant spread

1 eggplant
1 onion
1 cup celery
2 Tbsp. olive oil
1/4 lb. Greek olives, pitted
1 clove garlic
juice of 1 lemon
dash BioSalt or sea salt
dash cayenne

Bake eggplant. When done, remove skin. Do not lose any of the juice while peeling. Mix all ingredients in a blender and chill. Use on toast, crackers, or cut vegetables. Good for 4 days.

Millet-stuffed onions

12 medium-sized onions
1/2 cup millet, uncooked
2¹/₂ cups of water
dash of BioSalt or sea salt
2 cloves garlic, minced
1/2 cup mushrooms, sliced
1/2 cup celery, sliced
2 Tbsp. olive oil
1/2 cup chickpeas, cooked
1 cup almonds, grated
2 tsp. salty liquid seasoning
2 tsp. lemon juice
parsley for garnish

Hollow out insides of onions with an apple core, leaving bottoms intact and reserving insides. Steam hollowed-out onions until tender, reserving 3/4 cup of cooking liquid. Soak overnight and cook millet. Remove from heat and let stand, covered, for 10 minutes. Fluff with a fork. Finely chop reserved insides of onions. Sauté chopped onion, garlic, mushrooms, and celery for 15 minutes. Mix in millet and chickpeas and heat for about 5 minutes. Fill onions with millet mixture. Crush almonds with liquid seasoning and lemon juice in blender, then add reserved cooking liquid. Place mixture in a saucepan and heat, stirring constantly. Pour over stuffed onions, garnish with parsley, and serve. Serves 6

Quinoa casserole

- 1 cup quinoa, uncooked
- 1 Tbsp. olive oil
- 2 onions, thinly sliced
- 3 stalks celery, thinly sliced
- 1 cup chickpeas, cooked
- 5 cups water
- dash BioSalt or sea salt
- 2 cups broccoli, chopped
- parsley, minced, for garnish

Rinse and drain quinoa. Dry-roast quinoa in heavy skillet for 6 minutes, stirring constantly. Remove from heat. In 4 Tbsp. of water, sauté onions. Add celery, stirring often, and cook for about 5 minutes. Add chickpeas and water. Bring to a boil. Stir in quinoa and return to a boil. Reduce heat, cover, and simmer for 15 minutes. Add broccoli and continue to cook for 5 minutes. Add oil and BioSalt. While mixture is hot, press firmly into a 9-inch pan. Sprinkle with garnish, cut into squares, and serve. Serves 6

Sun seed paté

- 2 cups sunflower, pumpkin, or sesame seeds (soaked)
- 1 cup sprouts: alfalfa, onion, and/or radish
- 3 scallions
- 2 stalks celery or 1 cucumber
- 1/4 cup fresh parsley
- 3 Tbsp. lemon juice
- 1 Tbsp. dried basil
- 3 tsp. salty liquid seasoning
- dash of cayenne
- 1/2 cup carrots, grated

In Vita-Mix blender, blend all ingredients except carrots until slightly chunky. Put in a bowl and stir in carrots. Decorate with sprigs of parsley and sprinkles of cayenne. Serve with sprouted wheat or rye crackers. Serves 4

Falafel patties

In Vita-Mix blender, mix until smooth and creamy:
- 2 cups garbanzo beans, soaked 48 hours
- 1/2 cup sesame seeds, soaked 12 hours
- 1/2 cup wheatberry sprouts
- 1/4 cup fresh parsley
- 1 Tbsp. curry powder

1 Tbsp. basil
1 Tbsp. cumin powder
2 Tbsp. salty liquid seasoning
1/8 tsp. cayenne

Form into 2-inch balls. Place in dehydrator for 4 to 6 hours or until a crust has formed on outside, or use an oven at 100 degrees. The inside will be moist. To serve, place several patties on a grain crisp. Layer shredded lettuce and diced tomatoes and cucumber. Cover with Tahini Dressing and serve. Serves 2

Croquettes
2 cups lentil sprouts
1 clove garlic
1/4 Tbsp. cumin
1 cup poppy seeds (make into cheese by soaking overnight and grinding)
2 carrots, grated
1/4 cup scallion

Grind or mash lentil sprouts. Mix with other ingredients. Shape into croquettes and roll in poppy seeds. Serves 4

Tabouli
1 cup cracked wheat
1 cup finely chopped green onions, with tops
3 cups fresh parsley, chopped
3 cups fresh cilantro, chopped
4 finely chopped tomatoes
1/2 cup lemon juice
1/2 cup olive oil
Add cayenne, garlic, and kelp to taste

Soak cracked wheat overnight. Mix all remaining ingredients together. Add to soaked wheat. Allow to set for 3 hours so wheat can absorb flavors, then serve. Serves 4

Tabouli casserole
1 cup millet
1 cup cracked wheat

Soak overnight in 4 cups of water. Add remaining ingredients from previous recipe. Cook at low heat for 50 minutes and serve. Serves 8

Tasty legumes recipe
    2 cups garbanzos or any type of beans
    1/2 cup parsley, chopped
    1/2 cup cilantro, chopped
    1 cup onions, chopped
    1 cup carrots, chopped
    3 cloves garlic
    2 Tbsp. olive oil
    2 Tbsp. salty liquid seasoning
    pinch cayenne
    pinch powdered garlic
    pinch powdered kelp

Soak the beans overnight. Drain water; add fresh water and cook for 2 hours at low heat. Add parsley, cilantro, onions, carrots, and garlic while cooking. When ready to serve, add olive oil, liquid seasoning, and cayenne, garlic, and kelp to taste. Serve with brown rice or millet. Serves 8

ZOJIRUSHI NEUROFUZZY RICE COOKER

This multipurpose cooker for rice and other grains, steamed vegetables, and casseroles has some great features:

- Digital timer allows programming up to 13 hours in advance.
- Prepares delicious casseroles in just minutes.
- When food is perfectly cooked, it automatically stops cooking and switches to "warm."

cooking tip

For whole-grain cooking, press Menu and choose from the following settings:

- Regular—for brown rice, mixed rice, quinoa
- Softer—for white rice, porridge
- Harder—for fried rice, whole wheat, millet

Measure 1 cup of grain and 2 cups of water (rice or any other grain). You can add a portion of fresh chopped veggies or a packet of frozen veggies. Do not add any more water. Press the Cooking/Reheat button.

NEUROFUZZY COOKER RECIPES

These recipes were designed with this particular cooker in mind, but can be adjusted for stove top or crock pot.

Plain grain

1 cup grain: millet, quinoa, brown rice, whole wheat kernels, or steel-cut oats (Two different grains can be mixed.)
2 cups water

Add water to grain and turn switch to "regular." When cooking is perfectly done, cooker will switch to "keep warm" mode.
Serves 6

Potato casserole

3 onions, sliced
3 bell peppers, sliced
4 potatoes, sliced
4 sweet potatoes, sliced
1 cup water
1/2 cup Tahini Dressing or Healthful Green Dressing.
dash salty liquid seasoning
pinch cayenne
pinch BioSalt

Place half the onions, peppers, potatoes, and sweet potatoes in Neurofuzzy Cooker. Add the remaining onions, peppers, and potatoes. Add water. Add Tahini Dressing or Healthful Green Dressing. Turn cooker on "regular." Cook for 20 minutes. Unplug cooker and add liquid seasoning, cayenne, and BioSalt to taste.
Serves 4

Fast and tasty paella

1 cup grain
2 cups water
1 package frozen vegetables (green peas, corn, or mixed)
Optional: 1/2 to 1/3 cup Healthful Green Dressing, Tahini Dressing, or nut milk
fresh vegetables, chopped into bite-size pieces (onions, tomatoes, zucchini, carrots, sweet potatoes, etc.)
chicken, fish, or tofu, chopped into bite-size pieces

Place all ingredients in Neurofuzzy Cooker. Turn switch to "regular." When cooking is done, the cooker automatically switches to warming mode. Serves 8

Vegetable soup

2 quarts hot water
3 cups mixed chopped vegetables (onion, celery, potatoes, parsley, garlic, zucchini, etc.)

Cook on "regular" for 20 minutes in Neurofuzzy Cooker. Unplug cooker, and serve with salty liquid seasoning and cayenne. Serves 6

16 healthful sweets

Use healthful ingredients (no white flour or sugar please). Start experimenting with your palate. Your family will be glad you did!

Baked apples and pears

Filling:

1/2 cup dried apricots, chopped
1 cup almonds, ground
1 Tbsp. honey
1/2 tsp. cinnamon
1/2 banana
juice of 1 orange
juice of 1 lemon

To prepare filling: Soak dried apricots in warm water until soft, about 15 minutes. Combine apricots with remaining filling ingredients in mixing bowl. Set aside.

To assemble: Preheat oven to 400 degrees. Core 3 apples and 3 pears, and sprinkle with a little lemon juice. Press filling into cored area of each fruit. Place in lightly greased baking dish. Bake for 20 minutes or until tender but still firm. Remove fruit and let cool. Serves 6

Tofu-pita dessert

1 lb. cake of tofu
2 Tbsp. rice syrup or maple syrup
1 Tbsp. almond butter
4 to 6 pita pockets

Squeeze excess water out of the tofu. Blend tofu, rice syrup, and almond butter together. Fill pita pockets and lightly bake for a few minutes. Serves 4 to 6

Fruit salad

1 cup freshly squeezed orange juice
juice of 1/2 lemon
2 apples
2 pears
2 peaches
2 bananas
1/2 lb. grapes

Combine the orange juice and lemon juice in a large bowl. Add each fruit as you cut it, so that the juice in the bowl will keep it from discoloring. Cover the bowl with plastic wrap, and chill in the refrigerator for at least 2 hours before serving. Serves 6 to 8

Tofurella cheesecake

Crust:
1¹/₂ cups granola, crushed
3/4 cup graham cracker crumbs
1 Tbsp. melted raw butter
2 Tbsp. rice bran syrup
apple juice to moisten

Filling:
2 lb. Tofurella or other nondairy cheese substitute
1 tsp. vanilla
3 tsp. lemon juice
1/3 cup almond butter
6 Tbsp. rice bran syrup
dash cinnamon

Preheat oven to 350 degrees. Pulverize the granola and graham crackers together into very fine crumbs in a mixing bowl. Melt butter and rice syrup together over low heat, and add to crumbs. Add just enough apple juice to make mixture hold together. Press the crumb mixture evenly into a greased 9-inch pie pan. Bake for 10 minutes, remove, and cool completely. Reduce oven temperature to 325 degrees. Purée all of the filling ingredients in a blender until smooth. Pour the filling mixture into the crust, and bake at 325 degrees for 30 minutes. Turn the oven off, but leave the cheesecake in the oven for another 30 minutes before serving. Serves 8

Sesame crackers

2 cups water
1¹/₂ cups oil
2 tsp. BioSalt or sea salt
8 cups whole wheat flour
2 cups sesame seeds

Blend water, oil, and salt. Combine flour and sesame seeds with this mixture. Knead a little. Let rest 10 minutes. Roll out the dough and cut into cookie-size pieces. Bake at 350 degrees for 15 to 20 minutes. Makes 3 dozen.

Peanut butter apple sandwiches

1 medium apple
2 Tbsp. peanut butter or almond butter
2 Tbsp. soft or regular tofu, well drained
1 Tbsp. orange juice

Peel the apple while it is still whole. Slice apple crosswise into four to six slices. Cut out the core with a knife to make rings. In a bowl, mash together tofu and nut butter until almost smooth, then spread on one apple slice to make a sandwich. Repeat with remaining slices. Serves 1 to 2

Barbecued peaches with cream

6 fresh ripe peaches
1 Tbsp. melted butter
dash cinnamon
3 oz. kefir or yogurt
1/4 cup raw almonds

Wash peaches and cut in half. Remove pits. Brush with melted butter and barbeque or grill a few minutes on each side. Mix kefir and almonds in blender and serve as topping on peaches. Or top with Almond Cream or Tofu Cream below. Serves 4 to 6

Almond cream

1 cup raw almonds, soaked 48 hours
1/2 cup dates, pitted
1 tsp. vanilla extract
1 banana
1 cup water
2 Tbsp. lemon juice

Blend in blender until smooth and creamy.

Tofu cream

1 lb. firm tofu
2 bananas
2 Tbsp. honey
2 Tbsp. lemon juice
2 Tbsp. tahini or almond butter (optional)
1/2 tsp. vanilla

Blend in blender until smooth and creamy.

Healthful birthday treat—raggedy ann fruit salad

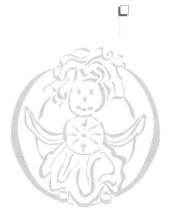

bananas—Arms
coconut—Hair
pears—Face
pineapple round—Chest
red cherries—Feet
carob candies—Nose, Eyes, Buttons
fruit salad covered with lettuce—Skirt

Serves 4 to 8

Apricot pie

Filling:
In bowl, soak for 6 hours:
2 cups dried apricots, cut in half
3 cups water

Blend in blender until smooth and creamy:
1 cup raw almonds, soaked 48 hours
10 dates
2 Tbsp. psyllium seed husks
water from soaked apricots

Place in bowl and stir in soaked apricots.

Pie Shell:
Blend until smooth and creamy:
2 cups raw almonds, not soaked
1/4 cup raisins
1/2 tsp. cinnamon
1–2 Tbsp. water

Press into a 9-inch pie pan. Pour apricot filling into pie shell. Chill and serve. Serves 6 to 8

17 herbs

Herbs are plants that have a healing quality, and herbalists see nature as a positive force in healing the body. In fact, many medical doctors recognize the benefits of natural methods of treatment with herbs. Scientific studies are being conducted to determine the basis for their effectiveness. Herbs provide the body with nutrients to help avoid disease and aid in the body's efforts to heal itself. Herbs can help balance the body's chemistry to protect against disease. They can be eaten fresh or made into teas, but most commonly are prepared into tinctures or dehydrated into capsules (for higher concentrations).

The following are some of the most common herbs traditionally used to foster good health and combat unhealthful conditions in the body. We recommend Nature's Sunshine and PRL herbs, available at many health food stores. Each container of herbs has a suggested dosage.

(This information is for educational purposes only. It is not intended to replace the services of any health professional.)

alfalfa

For pituitary gland, arthritis. Source of chlorophyll, highly nutritive. Alkalizes body rapidly, detoxifies body and liver.

algin

For detoxification, absorbs heavy metals such as lead and cadmium, able to remove radiation from the body.

barberry bark

For typhoid and jaundice. Improves appetite, acts as a laxative.

bayberry

Has been used for congestion in the nose and sinuses. It is extremely good for all female organs.

bee pollen

High in protein, it is considered an energy food. It also helps alleviate allergies.

black cohosh

Feeds and supports female system. Alleviates menstrual cramps, high blood pressure, spinal meningitis, poisonous bites. Relieves childbirth pain at delivery.

black currant oil

Builds blood. High in vitamin C, highly alkalizing, one of the highest sources of Gamma-Linolenic Acid (GLA).

black walnut

Cleanses parasites, expels tapeworms, relieves diarrhea.

blessed thistle

Strengthens the heart and lungs, takes oxygen to the brain.

blue cohosh

Regulates menstrual flow, makes childbirth easier. Relieves whooping cough, bronchial mucus, palpitations, high blood pressure, and spasms.

buckthorn

For rheumatism, gout, dropsy, skin disease.

burdock

Cleanser and blood purifier; used for acne, arthritis, boils, skin diseases, eczema.

butcher's broom

For varicose veins, hemorrhoids, phlebitis; anti-inflammatory. Helps kidneys.

capsicum

Catalyst for all herbs. Stops internal bleeding, aids circulation. Use with lobelia for nerves.

cascara sagrada

Relieves chronic constipation, gall stones; increases secretion of bile.

catnip

For convulsions in children. Used as sleep aid and to soothe nerves; calming in cases of insanity.

chamomile

Calms nerves, relieves toothache and muscle pain, helps stop smoking and use of alcohol.

chaparral

Cleanser and blood purifier. Relieves arthritis, acne, and boils.

chickweed

Bronchial cleanser, "eats" carbohydrates. Used to treat deafness, peritonitis.

comfrey

Blood cleanser. Used to treat ulcers, stomach, kidneys, bowel.

cornsilk

Used for kidney and bladder trouble, trouble with prostate gland in urinating, also for painful urination, and to prevent bed wetting.

damiana

For sexual impotency, reproductive organs. Used to overcome loss of nerve or loss of energy to limbs.

dandelion

Blood builder and purifier, liver cleanser. Very good for anemia.

dong quai

Corrects female problems, regulates blood pressure, cleans liver and blood.

echinacea

Antispasmodic. Prevents infection from spreading; used for skin problems, lymph glands, circulation, fevers.

evening primrose oil

For weight loss, high blood pressure, eczema, hot flashes, multiple sclerosis, arthritis, alcoholism.

eyebright

Aids vision and uppermost parts of the throat as far as the windpipe.

false unicorn

For miscarriage, problems with the female reproductive system, sterility, diabetes.

fennel

Has been used to eliminate colic in babies. Helps kill appetite, aids digestion.

fenugreek

Promotes healing fevers, moves mucus, lubricates intestines. Useful for the eyes, .

garlic

Has been used to emulsify cholesterol and loosen it from arterial walls. Effective in arresting intestinal putrefaction and infection.

ginger

Stimulates circulation.

ginseng

Provides support for the male hormone system, relieves prostate and stomach problems. Promotes longevity.

golden seal

Antibiotic, cleanser; relieves morning sickness. Cure-all-type herb.

gotu kola

Used for mental imbalance, blood pressure and energy imbalance, depression, nervous breakdown. Promotes longevity; strengthens the heart, memory, and brain.

grapevine

Used to relieve effects of smog; diuretic.

hawthorn berries

Have been used to dilate coronary blood vessels mildly and restore heart muscle wall.

hops

For insomnia, restlessness, shock. Decreases desire for alcohol.

ho-shu-wu

Promotes longevity.

horsetail

Heavy in silica, makes nails stronger. Has been used as a diuretic, helps with kidney stones.

hydrangea

For gallstones, kidney stones, bladder problems; diuretic.

juniper berries

Used for kidney or bladder problems related to pancreas and adrenal glands.

kelp

For thyroid, arteries, nails, hair loss. Cleanses radiation from body.

licorice root

Natural cortisone. Used for hypoglycemia, adrenal gland exhaustion, stress, colds.

mullein

Used for breathing problems, hay fever, glandular swelling, and as as a pain killer.

pau d'arco

Blood builder. Used for all types of cancer, diabetes, Hodgkin's disease, leukemia, psoriasis, ulcers, and more.

psyllium

Excellent colon cleanser, creates bulk, helps detoxification.

red clover

Blood purifier, relaxes the nerves and entire system.

rosehips

Has been used to fight infection and relieve stress.

sage

Prevents night sweats. Expels worms in children and adults. Stops bleeding of wounds and cleans old ulcers and sores.

sarsaparilla

Feeds male hormone system. Used for rheumatism, gout, psoriasis, and as an antidote for poison.

skullcap

Nerve tonic, strengthens heart. Used for rabies, hysteria, migraines.

slippery elm

Used for inflamed mucous membranes of the stomach, bowels, kidneys.

spirulina

High protein; increases energy, kills appetite. Balances RNA and DNA.

uva ursi

For diabetes, hemorrhoids, gonorrhea; supports kidneys, spleen, liver, pancreas.

valerian root

For nervous disorders, headache, muscle twitching, spasms. Promotes sleep.

white oak bark

Decongestant, blood purifier; used for asthma, hay fever, flu.

yucca

Has been used for rheumatoid and osteoid forms of arthritis.

18 home remedies

You will be surprised to learn about the effects of some common foods, such as garlic, onions, grapefruit, capsicum (cayenne), lemons, chlorophyll, and vitamin C.

NATURE'S ANTIBIOTICS

Garlic and onions, along with vitamin C, are the most important antibiotics in nature.

garlic

Garlic is the strongest natural antibiotic or bacteriostatic. Of all the natural home remedies, garlic has been used for the broadest number of diseases and disorders, and no doubt with the greatest success. It has no side effects. It destroys no blood cells; it inhibits the growth of tumor cells.

Garlic is useful for chronic disorders such as high blood pressure, kidney obstructions, hardening of the arteries, senility caused by alkaline toxins, accumulation of cholesterol, hepatitis, inflammation of the bladder, wounds, worms, ulcers, asthma, gastric and intestinal catarrh, sinusitis, and other ailments.

Garlic is a digestive stimulant, an intestinal antiseptic, and a glandular regulator. It is a good source of iodine and thus is beneficial for hypothyroid.

Use raw garlic on salads, sauté garlic with vegetables, use garlic powder for seasoning. Eat baked garlic, or take it in capsule form.

Garlic or onion tea

2 large bulbs (not cloves) of raw garlic
or 3 large onions
pinch cayenne (optional)
tomato juice (optional)

Cut garlic or onions crosswise into a quart and a half of water (they need not be peeled). Cook until tender (do not use aluminum cookware). Strain and drink a cup of this tea every 20 minutes. Onion or garlic tea is almost tasteless, but very effective. Cayenne makes it more effective, and tomato juice may be added.

onions

Onions have the same antibiotic effect as garlic but are not as strong.

Onion cough syrup
2 cups onion, chopped
1/2 cup honey

Combine onion with honey. Keep the mixture warm by placing it in a hot-water bath for 3 hours, and then strain. Take 1 teaspoon of the mixture as needed for cough.

steamed onion poultice

For chest decongestion. The steamed onion tea can be applied hot with a cheese cloth over the chest as a poultice to produce chest decongestion. Leave it on for 20 minutes. Repeat 3 times daily.

grapefruit—antibiotic, bacteriostatic

The bitter tea of grapefruit relieves aching and the discomfort associated with acute infectious diseases. The fruit is a natural antibiotic with no side effects. Cooking garlic or onions with the grapefruit makes it doubly effective. You cannot make the grapefruit tea taste worse by adding garlic or onions, so why not combine them?

Grapefruit and Epsom salt packs have been used with excellent results for a wide variety of disorders, such as colitis, hay fever, bronchial and lung diseases, sore throat, erysipelas, neuritis, mumps, bruises, cuts, abscesses, boils and carbuncles, and blood poisoning.

Grapefruit and garlic tea
2 grapefruits
2 large bulbs garlic
1$\frac{1}{2}$ quarts water
pinch cayenne (optional)

Remove the yellow grapefruit peel with a potato peeler, and cut the fruit thinly. Add grapefruit and peeled garlic to water. Cook until very bitter, about 20 minutes. Drink a cup of this tea every 20 minutes. By the time the tea is gone, the infection is usually gone too. I use this along with enemas.

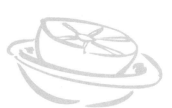

Grapefruit and epsom salt packs

1 whole grapefruit
1 to 1¹/₂ pints water
1 cup Epsom salts

Grind the grapefruit or cut it fine. Add it to the water, and boil slowly for 15 minutes. Strain. Add all the Epsom salt; it will dissolve in the water. Wet cheese cloths in the hot solution and apply locally for 20 minutes.

capsicum (cayenne, red pepper)—antibiotic, bacteriostatic

Cayenne equalizes the circulation and has an influence on the whole system. It promotes elimination through the skin when sweat baths or Epsom salt baths are taken. Cayenne is especially healing to the mucous membrane of the throat and the entire alimentary canal. It is specific for sore throat, diphtheria, influenza, and colds. It may be added to the teas mentioned above (Onion and Garlic Tea or Grapefruit and Garlic Tea), or it may be taken in capsules every 2 hours, with food or drink.

acne

All of the following treatments are helpful for acne:

1. Acne may be caused by a deficiency of vitamin B_{12} and folic acid. These nutrients are found in molasses and nutritional food yeast. Twelve tablets of high-potency nutritional food yeast daily will supply these nutrients in abundance. We recommend KAL brand.
2. Honey draws pus from boils and carbuncles rapidly, and can also help in treating severe acne. Garlic oil may be added to the honey and the mixture applied at bedtime.
3. Vitamin F (essential fatty acids) is necessary for all healthy internal and external tissue. It is found in lecithin.
4. A mixture of bentonite clay and water applied to acne is very effective.
5. Animal fats and fried food, white sugar and white flour products, chocolate, soft drinks, coffee, tea, and tobacco should be eliminated from the diet.
6. Vegetables and vegetable juices and broths, fruits and fruit juices are cleansing, alkaline, nonmucus-forming foods that help to prevent acne.

arteriosclerosis (hardening of the arteries)

Dandelion, spinach, and beet tops have been used for hardening of the arteries. Eat them in salads or steamed.

arthritis

Alfalfa seed tea, made by simmering a tablespoon of seed in a quart of water, is specific for arthritis. Alfalfa contains over 50 nutrients, and the seed is more potent than the leaves.

bladder, kidney, and ureter inflammation

Peach leaf tea will eliminate pain and discomfort and heal the entire urinary tract. Dandelion root tea increases the flow of urine and activates the liver. Boil 1 tsp. of dandelion root in a cup of water for 2 minutes.

Peach leaf tea

1 quart water
4 tsp. dry peach leaves, somewhat crushed.
2 cloves garlic (optional)

Stir the peach leaves into the water. Cover and simmer for 10 to 15 minutes; strain and drink a cup four times daily. Garlic may be simmered with the leaves.

bone fractures

Lemons contain the vitamin C and calcium needed for mending bones. Comfrey is also noted for bone mending and is available in capsule form.

burns

- Peppermint oil or natural oil of wintergreen, applied straight or in honey, will relieve the pain of burns immediately. Either of these can be added to any dressing that will stay on.
- Dr. Edwin Wisdom tells us that alum powder, made into a paste with honey or water, will act as an antiseptic in burns.
- Scars from burns become almost invisible when treated with honey. Vitamin E may be added to the honey.

dental shock and weakness

As little as 500 mg of vitamin C given orally prevents shock and weakness after dental extractions.

Chlorophyll capsules (8 or 10) taken before and after dental extraction will prevent all soreness, shock, and pain, and the gums heal quickly.

hot flashes

A daily enema and herbal laxative to cleanse the bowel, and kelp tablets daily, will relieve hot flashes.

menstruation—painful

Toxins absorbed into the tissues of the cervix and uterus from the rectum cause inflammation and painful menstruation. Detoxification and rebuilding are indicated. The following herbs are helpful: blue cohosh, black cohosh, and squaw vine available from Nature Sunshine, one of the largest and oldest herbal companies.

kidney stones

Beet tops and beet roots have a dissolving effect on kidney stones. They may be purchased in tablet form at any health store. Include them in salads, steamed vegetables, and juices. They are a good food for your liver.

The Liver is one of the most important organs of the body, because it is the detoxification organ. It produces more than 13,000 different chemicals and 2,000 different enzymes that your body needs. Your liver could be functioning at 20 percent and doctors will not detect that you have a liver problem. Anything you could do to benefit your liver is a plus for your health. Do liver flushes (p. 38) three times a year, eat steamed artichokes with a dressing of olive oil and lemon juice. The water from the artichokes is really bitter, but drinking it is like medication for your liver. Also, include steamed asparagus often in your diet with a dressing of olive oil and lemon juice. Drinking the water from the asparagus is very cleansing, good for the liver and kidneys; it contains vitamin B_{17} and laetrile, provides protection against cancer, and is a great diuretic.

stings—insects

Vitamin C (500 mg) mixed in 1 Tbsp. honey relieves the pain of ant, wasp, yellow jacket, bee, and hornet stings. Remove the stinger before applying. If you have nothing else, you can mix some dirt or clay with water and apply the mud to the sting. The pain will soon be gone.

warts

A wart is a localized, benign (nonmalignant) hypertrophy of the skin.

Common warts are usually easy to remove by application of a piece of cotton saturated with castor oil or vitamin E. Hold the saturated cotton in place with an adhesive bandage during the night and, if possible, during the day as well. The wart usually falls off after a few days.

Some warts will not budge with this local application. If this is the case, eat cooked asparagus (a member of the grass family), which contains vitamin B_{17}. Four tablespoons of asparagus eaten daily for two months usually removes warts. The bandage described above may also be used along with the asparagus.

INJURIOUS EFFECTS OF TEA AND COFFEE

Dr. Edward Smith demonstrated that "Caffeine increases the ability to work, but an increase in fatigue follows. The effect is exhaustion of the cells."

Dr. H. H. Rugby said, "Caffeine is a genuine poison. It tends to be habit-forming. It causes permanent disease of the heart in its structural function, and of the nervous system also."

Caffeine tends to raise blood pressure. Dr. Kellogg of Battle Creek Sanitarium observed that the everyday intake of coffee raised abnormal blood pressure 20 to 40 points. Coffee makes your body and blood very acid. Your goal is to be more alkaline.

The tannic acid in tea is a powerful astringent. It suppresses the digestive juices and causes indigestion. It precipitates pepsin. Dr. Roberts found that tea destroys the action of saliva, and prevents digestion of carbohydrates in the stomach. It is best to avoid coffee and tea altogether (Theodore A. Baroody, *Alkalize or Die*).

suggested reading
Baroody, Theodore A.
Alkalize or Die
Holographic Health Press, Waynesville, NC, 1991

General Index

Recipe Index

Resources

FINDING ORGANIC PRODUCE

Look for health food stores, co-ops, and CSAs in your Yellow Pages.

If you have internet access, the following Web sites will direct you to local organic food retailers, coops, home delivery services, and even restaurants:

LocalHarvest.org
Organic Consumers Association,
http://www.organicconsumers.org/
Organic Trade Association Countrywide Organic Retailer Page, www.theorganicpages.com
Vegetarian Source Online, www.vegsource.com

Visit the Web sites of the following large health-food-store chains to find a location near you:

Whole Food Stores, www.wholefoods.com
Wild Oats, www.wildoats.com
Trader Joe's, www.traderjoes.com

Many large U.S. supermarket chains now have a good selection of organic produce and groceries, including:

Albertson's
P & C
Shop N' Save
Shop Rite
WalMart
Wegman's

Regional health-food-store chains service entire areas in the United States:

Illinois
Fruitful Yield Stores www.fruitfulyield.com
New York/Connecticut
Mrs. Green's Natural Food Markets
Washington
PCC Natural Markets

Organic Home Delivery Services
http://www.organickitchen.com/markets.html has a listing of organic home delivery services and organic grocers by region, including Canada, the United Kingdom, and the United States.
Boxed Greens Organic Produce, Inc., toll free at 888-588-8107, www.boxedgreens.com
Diamond Organics, mail order by phone toll free, 1-888-ORGANIC (674-2642)
Door to Door Organics, home delivery and UPS throughout New England, (215) 794-9828
Farm Fresh To You (800.796.6009), www.farmfreshtoyou.com, in the San Francisco Bay and greater Sacramento areas
Organic Connection, Westchester/Putnam/Fairfield counties of New York and Connecticut, www.organicconnection.net

Canadian Organic Retailers
Whole Foods
many local stores and health food stores

United Kingdom Organic Produce Retailers
Sainsbury's
Fresh and Wild
Planet Organic

Australian Organic Retailers
DynamicOrganics.com
GreenGrocer.com.au
WorldWholeFoods.com for info on stores that carry organic food in Australia

RECOMMENDED SUPPLEMENTS

Available at health food stores unless otherwise noted.

Chlorophyll and Green Foods
Blue Green Magma (**Dynamic Fitness**)
Essential Light (**We Care**)*
Green Magma (**Dr. Hagiwara's**)
Kyogreen (**Wakanuga**)
Power Green (**We Care** brand)*
Spirulina (**Earthwise**)
Super Blue Green (**Cell Tech Products**)
Super Green Formula (**NOW Foods**)

Enzyme Supplements
Food N-Zymes (**We Care** brand)*
Plant Enzymes (**NOW Foods**)
Primagest (www.drmickhall.com)
Ultrazyme Plus (**Silver Water**, Rochester, WA 98579;
   telephone: 360-458-2562)

Fiber Supplements
Detox Drink (**We Care** brand)*
Henry's Organic Internal Cleanser
   (www.greenlineorganic.com)
Intestinal Cleanser—Sonne's #9 (**Sonne's Organic
   Foods, Inc.**)
Psyllium Husk Powder (**NOW Foods**)
Super Seed (**Garden of Life Nutritional Products**)

Food and Supplements Containing Beneficial Bacteria
Kefir, Kefir Starter, goat and sheep yogurts, and sauer-
   kraut are all whole-food sources of probiotics and
   are available in most health food stores
Kyo-dophilus (**Wakunaga/Kyolic Products**)
Lactobacillus Bifidus (**Euglan Topfer Forte**)
NutriDophilus (www.drmickhall.com)
Super Acidophilus (**Twin Labs**)

Goat's Whey
Goatein (**Garden of Life**)
Goat's Whey (**Mt. Capra Wholefood Nutritionals**)
My Whey (**We Care** brand)*

Lecithin
Lecithin granules, gel caps, liquid (**NOW Foods**)
Pure Lecithin (**We Care** brand)*

Parasite Cleansers
Para Cleanse (**Nature's Sunshine Products**,
   www.naturessunshine.com)
Para Gone (**ReNew Life Formulas**)

Stablized Rice Bran Solubles
Life Solubles (**Integris**, www.integriscorp.com)

Stevia Sweeteners
Stevia Extract (**NOW Foods**)
Alcohol-free Stevia with Vegetable Glycerite (**NOW
   Foods**)
Stevia Clear (**Sweet Leaf**)

Table Salt Replacements
BioSalt, a nutritionally balanced salt alternative
   (www.wecarespa.com, www.caycecures.com, and
   through select health food stores)
Herbamare, Trocomare , an organic herb and salt blend
   (**A. Vogel**)
Liquid Aminos (**Bragg's**)
My-Protein, a nonfermented, liquid salty seasoning
   high in minerals (**We Care**)*
Quick Sip (**Jensens**)
Organic Tamari, wheat free (**Eden**)

KITCHEN MACHINES

Vita Mix Total Nutrition Center
   (800-848-2649, www.vitamix.com) available through
   We Care Spa and many health-product retailers
   (see Chapter 11)

Zojirushi Neurofuzzi Rice Cooker
   available through many online retailers
   (www.asiachi.com, www.wecarespa.com)
   and select department stores (see Chapter 15)

* Distributed by: **We Care Holistic Health Spa & Retreat**, Desert Hot Springs, CA 92241. Information: 1-800-888-2523,
www.wecarespa.com.

More Great Titles from Vital Health Publishing

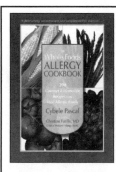

The Whole Foods Allergy Cookbook

Gourmet Recipes for the Food Allergic Family

by Cybele Pascal

ISBN: 1-890612-45-6 $18.95

The first gourmet cookbook to eliminate ALL eight allergens responsible for 90% of food allergies. 200 recipes. No dairy, eggs, wheat, soy, peanuts, tree nuts, fish or shellfish or even refined sugar in any recipe!

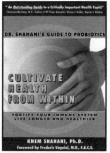

Cultivate Health From Within

Dr. Shahani's Guide to Probiotics

by Khem Shahani, Ph.D.

ISBN: 1-890612-42-1 $13.95

Find out how to supplement your diet to alleviate anxiety, produce natural antibiotic-like agents, assist digestion of fats and carbohydrates, improve HDL/LDL ratios, fight fungal, yeast and Candida infections.

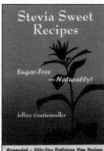

Stevia Sweet Recipes

Sugar Free – Naturally!

by Jeffrey Goettemoeller

ISBN: 1-890612-13-8 $13.95

168 stevia recipes. Stevia is all-natural, non-glycemic and proven safe! Great for diabetics and a healthy alternative to refined sugar or artifical sweeteners!

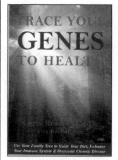

Trace Your Genes To Health

Use Your Family Tree to Overcome Chronic Disease

by Chris Reading, M.D.

ISBN: 1-890612-23-5 $15.95

Clear explanation of how to prevent and carefully manage health problems through tracing family health trees and following tailored nutritional guidelines.

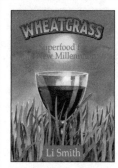

Wheatgrass

Superfood for a New Millenium

by Li Smith

ISBN: 1-890612-10-3 $10.95

A great book on growing and juicing your own wheatgrass, the benefits of wheatgrass juice, juicing and a fresh food diet, plus fabulous power drink recipes!

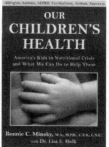

Our Children's Health

America's Kids in Nutritional Crisis And What We Can Do to Help Them

By Bonnie C. Minsky, M.P.H.

ISBN: 1-890612-27-8 $15.95

Symptoms, causes and natural treatments for ADHD, Allergies, Asthma and Weight Problems. Guidelines to creating a healthy environment for children, recipes for healthy eating, supplementation and more!

Facets of a Diamond
Reflections of a Healer

By John Diamond, M.D.

ISBN: 1-890995-17-7 $16.95

"Diamond needs to be more broadly read and appreciated for the depth and breadth of his knowledge of the human healing process."
Richard A. Lippin, M.D.

The Healer
Heart and Hearth

By John Diamond, M.D.

ISBN: 1-890995-22-3 $13.95

An incredible and original understanding of the role of the healer and of the sufferer representing the culmination of John Diamond's forty plus years in traditional and holistic therapies.

The Cancer Handbook
What's Really Working

By Lynne McTaggart

ISBN: 1-890612-18-9 $12.95

Compiled by the editors of the bestselling alternative health U.K. newsletter:
What Doctors Don't Tell You
www.wddty.com

GMO Free
Exposing the Hazards of Biotechnology To Ensure the Integrity of Our Food Supply

By Mae-Wan Ho, Ph.D.

ISBN: 1-890612-37-5 $10.95

The strongest published case for the banning of GMO's worldwide, written by a leading scientist and the respected 600 member independent science panel.

All Vital Health and Enhancement Books titles are available to the trade through Baker & Taylor, Ingram, Lotus Light, New Leaf, Nutri-Books, Partner's West and NOW Foods.

International: AU: Brumby Books, NZ: Peaceful Living, SA: New Horizons, UK: Deep Books. For Special Orders, Inquiries, or if you cannot locate a book at your local retailer, contact:

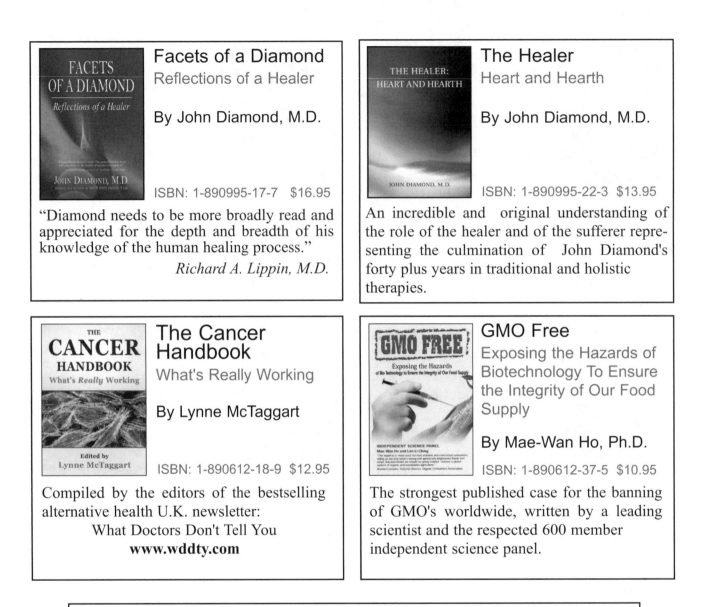

VITAL HEALTH PUBLISHING/ENHANCEMENT BOOKS

34 Mill Plain Road, Danbury, CT 06811
203-794-1009   1-877-VIT-BOOKS
www.vitalhealthbooks.com

We Care Holistic Health Spa

The 'health spa to the stars' in Desert Hot Springs, California

We Care Holistic Health Spa is a holistic fasting and spiritual retreat, providing unique programs designed for personal transformation, enhancing body, mind and spirit in a serene desert oasis.

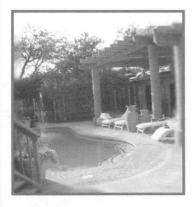
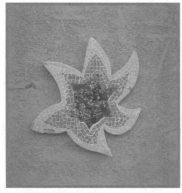

Diet and Nutrition

The Detoxification and Nutrition Program is central to the We Care Program.

Includes:
- Liquid Diet
- Supervised Fasting
- Diet Management
- Nutrition and Food Preparation Instruction

Results include increased energy, mental alertness, improved skin tone and elimination of dependencies on alcohol, caffeine, nicotine.

Body Treatments

We Care body treatments accelerate the cleansing process by relieving blockages in energy flow.

Treatments include:
- Colonics
- Reflexology
- Acupressure
- Massage Therapies
- Raindrop therapy,
- Body scrubs to open clogged pores and remove dead skin allowing the sweat glands to work more effectively in eliminating toxins.

Psychological and Spiritual Balancing

The We Care Program includes daily activities to enhance psychological and spiritual balance.

Daily offerings include:
- Yoga, meditation
- Breath work
- Desert walks
- Labyrinth
- Medicine wheel

All of these aspects of the program complement each other to yield optimal results in one's overall health and psycho-spiritual balance.

Detox ◆ Revitalize ◆ Cleanse ◆ Renew

Visit We Care Spa

www.wecarespa.com   1-800-888-2523